The 5 Habits of Healthy People

The 5 Habits of Healthy People

A simple five-step blueprint to living a long and healthy life

MARK CHAVEZ M.D.

THE HEALTH MD

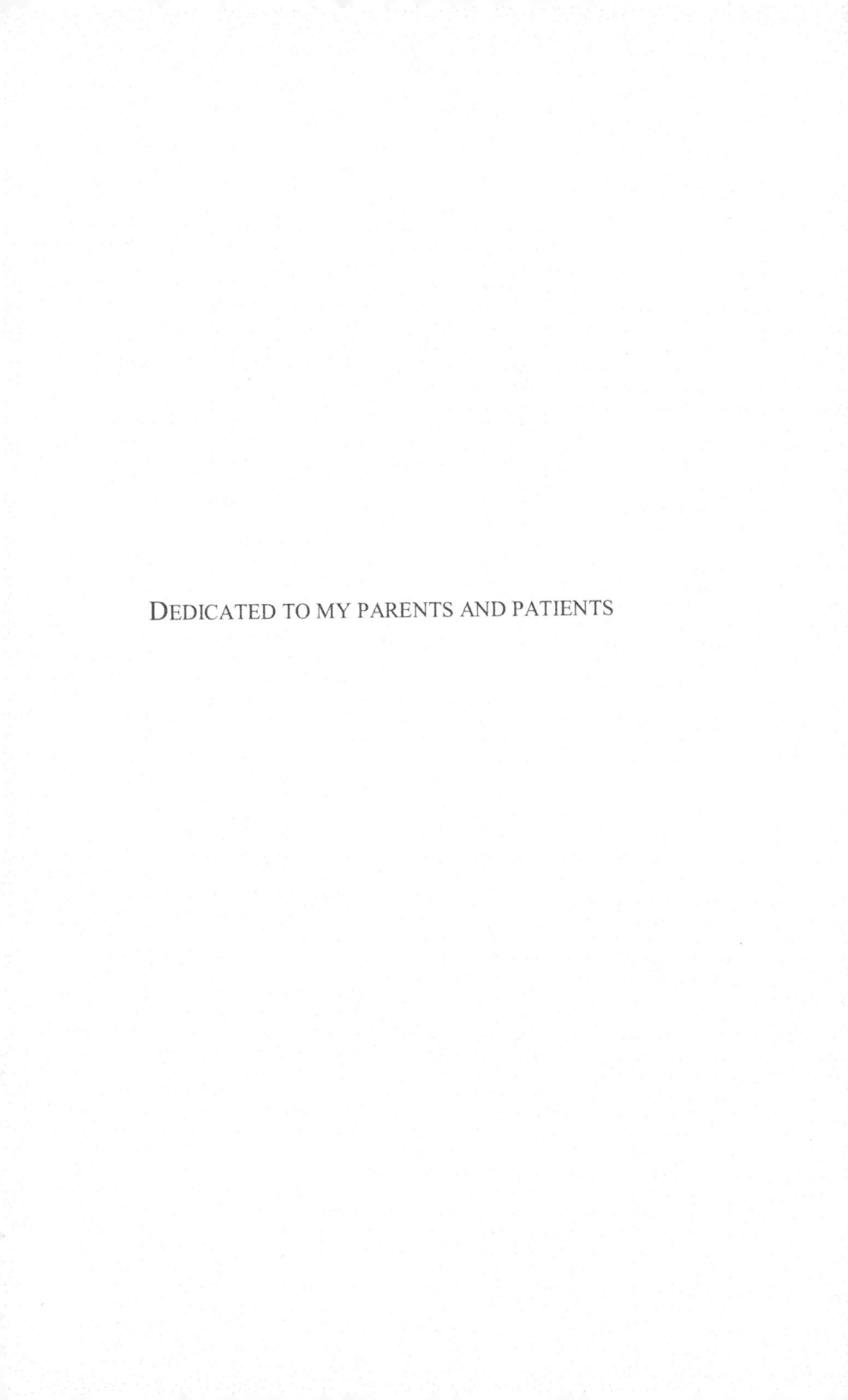

DEDICATED TO MY PARENTS AND PATIENTS

TABLE OF CONTENTS

Why You Should Read This Book

Did you know the current health-care system in this country was designed to treat disease, not to keep people healthy? In fact, health care was originally called "sick care" in its early days. Unfortunately, at its core, that hasn't changed. So why should we expect the health-care system to do something it wasn't designed to do?

But here's the good news. If you want to get and stay healthy, there is a way. Developing five keystone habits will take you there. These habits are part of a different way to look at health care. That's why, as a practicing physician, I wrote this book: to offer a program of health that actually works and that can be used throughout all stages of life.

The 5 Habits of Healthy People™ is for the person who wants to live a long and healthy life, free of reliance on the medical system. Reading this book, you can expect to take away simple, actionable advice to use immediately without needing any science background or medical training to understand it.

The 5 Habits™ were born from my own self-experimentation, my experience with patients, and my studies in the fields of science, fitness, nutrition, chemistry, medicine, and the psychology of habit-building. Keystone habits, as coined by the best-selling author Charles Duhigg, who wrote the book *The Power of Habit: Why We Do What We Do in Life and Business*, are key habits that, when maintained, will have a profound effect on your life, oftentimes in unforeseeable ways.[1]

The 5 Habits are keystone habits. After reading this book, you will have the knowledge and practical steps to create an action plan for yourself using The 5 Habits blueprint. Consistent practice will transform your life in ways that you never believed possible.

What This Book Is Not

This book is not medical advice, nor is it a callout to never go to the doctor's office. When you have an urgent health issue or medical emergency, don't hesitate to go to your doctor or the ER! Doctors and the health-care system can be lifesaving in many situations. This book doesn't focus on acute health issues or emergencies. It's not a replacement for conventional medicine.

Rather, it's focused on improving daily and long-term health by executing important habits consistently. It's also a call to action for us physicians and medical professionals to step up and educate ourselves in greater depth in topics relevant to health, fitness, and nutrition, or at the very least, to direct patients to trusted resources where they can get this information.

We've found many ways to lengthen our life-span in terms of technologically advanced treatments, but we've dropped the ball on teaching people and providing them with the tools to live longer with a higher quality of life. This is best done by teaching healthy ways of living and by rewarding healthy behaviors. The objective of the current system is to profit from sickness. It's time for a new system that rewards health and incentivizes providers to keep people healthy.

Remember, your health is your greatest asset, and investing in yourself is the best investment you can make.

So are you ready to take control?

If the answer is yes, read on.

A Better Model of Health Care

Since the purpose of the current health-care system has been to serve people who fall ill, an alternate but parallel health-care system is needed to help millions of people avoid societally borne diseases. This system would be, in fact, a true system of health care. It would train doctors to optimize health and human potential, not simply wait until people get sick to treat their illnesses with medications and procedures.

Scientific knowledge and medical advances have conquered many of the diseases that were prevalent in the past. Viruses and infectious agents, including fleas, mosquitoes, and ticks, combined with unclean environments, produced major epidemics and public health emergencies. Cholera and smallpox, for example, killed millions of people prior to the development of vaccines and antibiotics and the understanding and acceptance of germ theory.

Today, with all the advances of science and technology, our medical system has become good at diagnosing and treating complex diseases and developing important vaccines and surgical procedures that have lengthened life-spans and eradicated many diseases in the developed world. However, these advances are very different from the practices needed to manage, prevent, and reverse the diseases of a technologically dependent society.

Physicians have traditionally served as the gatekeepers of our nation's health. But their medical training focuses primarily on pathology (illness). They're trained to diagnose and treat disease by administering medicines, performing procedures, and ordering various tests.

They're not trained to keep people healthy including themselves. This is why there are so many unhealthy doctors. This is crazy, as many of the top killers in the United States are still largely preventable diseases. We know the list: heart disease, cancer, stroke, and diabetes. Most of these diseases are avoidable with simple and inexpensive behavioral modifications. No amount of investment into technology or pharmaceutical research can replace the value and return on investment that preventive actions and education provide.

Imagine this: If your doctor actually sat down with you, listened carefully to your thoughts and concerns, and then partnered with you to create a plan to address your concerns and optimize your health, how great would that be!

The Medical "System" Is Not What It Seems

The truth is that your health is simply not the focus for most doctors. They're trained to find illnesses with tests and treat it or manage it with drugs. Furthermore, managing medical conditions is a highly profitable business over time. In business terms, this is known as the *lifetime value of the customer*. By managing health conditions instead of curing them, the lifetime value of the customer to the medical and pharmaceutical industries skyrockets over time (with some exceptions). It is from sick people that large medical and pharmaceutical industries continue to profit.

———————————————— BASELINE HEATLH ————————————————

OPTIMIZED HEALTH   SUB-OPTIMAL HEALTH   PRE-DISEASE   DISEASE

....   HEALTH   ....   MEDICAL   ....
            CARE   CARE

As this image shows, on the spectrum of disease to health, the medical system lies in the realm of the pre-disease and disease states. It rarely crosses over to the realm of health. Many of these chronic diseases are man-made diseases that coincide with the mass production and incorporation of processed sugars and unnatural fats and other chemicals into the American diet. Conditions such as diabetes, metabolic syndrome, high blood pressure, and some autoimmune diseases, as well as many joint and musculoskeletal disorders, are for the most part man made.

It took me many years to really see and understand how the system operates. When I did, I was extremely disheartened. I came to see what my role was as a medical provider. I was a distributor and consumer of products and services in the form of tests, procedures, and medications that much of the time offered little to no meaningful benefit to my patients. Over the last 15 years of practicing medicine, I have come to realize just how dysfunctional and inefficient the medical system is.

What I Wasn't Taught in Medical School

During their first year of medical school, new medical students take the Hippocratic oath (or some version of the Hippocratic oath), which swears them to do everything in their power to serve the patient and never knowingly harm them. For four years during medical school, we are funneled through hundreds of lectures and numerous labs to learn about "normal" and diseased states. We're taught ways to diagnose and treat disease using various tests, medications, and procedures.

What we are not taught is the power that diet, exercise, mind-set, sleep, and emotions have in preventing and reversing disease. Furthermore, we are not taught how the medical system functions, and we aren't told that we will be working within a system that doesn't have the same goals for the patients as we did when we idealistically chose to become "healers."

Soon after becoming a physician, I felt ill equipped to provide my patients with any real value, as my training did not cover health, nutrition, or fitness. When patients came to me seeking advice about these issues, I was not able to offer much insight about the things that they really cared about. I was ashamed that I didn't have good advice or answers for them.

But now I do.

How Did I Get to The 5 Habits?

The 5 Habits of Healthy People was born out of the perfect storm in my own life.

I was working long hours as a physician with a constantly changing schedule that that left me tired, sleep deprived, depressed, and moody. As a result, I let my weight balloon by more than 60 pounds. I didn't exercise, became unfit and stressed out, and kept a terrible diet. I was ashamed of how badly I had let my health go and felt like a hypocrite advising patients that they should live healthier and make better choices.

Around the same time, my father, who is a body builder, sustained a devastating nerve injury to both his hands while undergoing surgery. This nerve injury left him unable to fully close his hands and grip things.

After my father was injured, I realized that many of my patients had the same issue with grip strength, which also renders them unable to do strength-based exercise using weight.

I understood that lack of regular resistance exercise is the main cause of many of the musculoskeletal problems I see on a daily basis. After interviewing hundreds of people, I learned that most people didn't really understand the importance of doing resistance exercise. I also realized that most of the chronic pain I was seeing in my patients such as back pain, shoulder pain, knee pain, and neck pain was due to muscle weakness and imbalances. Most of the people who suffer from these conditions have lost significant muscle mass, which has led to weak and imbalanced joints. Virtually all of this can be fixed with a program of regular resistance exercise.

Most back, shoulder, knee and neck pain is due to muscle weakness and imbalance. Resistance exercise could make all this pain disappear.

Building on this realization, I shifted my focus back to my own health and implemented The 5 Habits into my life. By doing this, I have transformed my health and lost over 60 pounds, and I've remained at my ideal weight for the last seven years. In the process of doing this, I've completed 11 marathons, including the Boston Marathon in 2016. Health is now, and will always be, a top priority in life, and I make time for it every day. I have been able to do this is by utilizing *The 5 Habits of Healthy People* blueprint.

So can you.

The Keystone Habits

Throughout this book, I will walk you through each of The 5 Habits, explaining the importance of each and how integrating them into your life will positively affect your health, regardless of how healthy or unhealthy you are now.

The 5 Habits of Healthy People blueprint is a simple five-step method for taking back your health and maintaining it for life.

Consistent application of these five simple habits in your daily routine will be rewarded with good health, a strong mind and body, and endless possibilities to live an exceptional life.

Some of these ideas might not be new to you. For example, most kids can accurately describe what behaviors are important to be healthy: "Eat, nap, sleep well, play, run, and have fun every day." When it comes down to it, health really is just a series of habits that we put in place in our everyday lives.

If It's So Simple, Why Is It Such a Struggle?

The United States is faced with a big task of providing health care for a diverse group of Americans with a wide range of chronic and often complicated health conditions.[2] As physicians get more frustrated with the direction of the medical system, many are seeking alternatives and are looking to leave medicine altogether.

High-profile physicians like Dr. William Davis are spreading their message through online outlets, including podcasts and books like his book, *Undoctored: Why Health Care Has Failed You and How You Can Become Smarter Than Your Doctor*.[3] Others are launching new ventures to bring doctors closer to their patients through concierge services and by encouraging patients to use activity trackers and other smart devices to equip themselves with ways to access their own health information and take responsibility for their own health.

These actions are a good next step, but first, we have to stop making ourselves sick! Despite the variety of viewpoints and proposed solutions, many of the top diseases in the United States are still largely preventable. It is worth repeating that these diseases are avoidable with straightforward behavior changes that can be learned and adopted as simple habits. No amount of investment in technology or pharmaceutical research can replace the value and return on investment that preventive actions and education provide.

Second, medical schools should also teach physicians how to get and keep people healthy, not just how to diagnose and treat people after they have fallen ill. Right now, they're doing an abysmal job. In fact, I often recommend that friends and family avoid asking their doctors for health advice, as the advice they get from their physician oftentimes leaves them more confused than ever, not to mention that many physicians themselves set a terrible example. They're often unhealthy themselves and lead lives of stress, poor sleep, and terrible eating habits.

This shouldn't be a surprise. In my entire four years of medical school, we only had a single one-hour lecture on nutrition! Furthermore, I don't remember having any instruction on exercise or fitness. If this is the type of education that our medical professionals are getting, then we need to rethink who the experts are in health and wellness.

As a country, we spend far less on preventive education and care than other countries.[4] While preventive care isn't as profitable in the short term as fancy pharmaceuticals, high-tech procedures, and extensive laboratory testing of the current business model of our health-care system, if we take a long-term perspective, we can see that a healthier nation is a much more valuable and profitable nation.

The 5 Habits of Healthy People is a blueprint for healthy living. It was created to provide a simple way to achieve and maintain lasting health for anybody who wants to live a long, healthy life, while bypassing the doctor's office. The goal of this book is to give you the tools that will help to keep you from relying on the health-care system for as long as possible and will give you the knowledge and insight to take control of your health.

Now let's get started!

THE 5 HABITS OF HEALTHY PEOPLE

These five habits were born out of my experiences with my own health; my patients; and my training, education, and studies over the last 30 years. I am both excited and happy to share them with you here.

Now let's dive into Habit #1!

Chapter 1

Habit #1: Daily Resistance Exercise

Over the years, I've asked hundreds of patients what they do for exercise. Walking is the most common answer I get. Other answers I get include walking the dog around the block every day or taking a walk after dinner. Most people understand the importance of doing some regular cardio-based activity to stay healthy.

Almost nobody mentions resistance exercise, also known as strength training. Even if they understand its importance, they don't know much about it. This is one of the paradoxes in our modern society of ease and convenience. To maintain health, it is necessary to do *both* cardio and resistance exercise on a regular basis. In fact, it is my belief that resistance exercise is at least as important as cardio-based exercise, if not more important.

The importance of doing resistance exercise for optimal health isn't a new idea. In the classic 1977 documentary *Pumping Iron*, a 28-year-old Arnold Schwarzenegger catapulted the sport of bodybuilding into public spotlight. After seeing Arnold with his almost superhuman physique, the average person was intimidated into thinking that lifting weights was something they couldn't or shouldn't do.[5]

Schwarzenegger later spoke about his desire to change the fitness industry and people's misconceptions about exercising with weight. He encouraged average people to lift weights, eat well, and live healthy at a time when lifting weights was thought to be dangerous to your health.[6]

Despite the growing acceptance of resistance exercise into the mainstream, the "gym rat" stereotype of bodybuilders using heavy iron weights has persisted.

In general, the average person does not adopt resistance exercise into their daily routine for one or both of the following reasons:

1. They don't really understand the benefits for them.
2. They don't know how to do resistance exercise safely and effectively.

Why Resistance Exercise?

There's a reason that the first of The 5 Habits is daily resistance exercise. The benefits of resistance exercise are numerous and backed by loads of science. Healthy people share this habit.

Simply put, daily resistance exercise is necessary to maintain a properly functioning body over time.

Daily resistance exercise helps you maintain a properly functioning body.

Resistance exercise is any form of exercise that applies a load or a force to your muscles and skeletal system that causes the muscles to contract in order to counter the load. It is a positive stressor that causes the muscles and bones to adapt to the load by growing stronger.

This beneficial stress also keeps tendons and other connective tissue strong and elastic, which guards against injury and stabilizes joints. Bone also requires this type of positive stress to remain dense and strong and prevent osteoporosis. As people age, they naturally lose muscle mass over time unless something is done to counter this progressive muscle loss. Most people's activity levels also tend to decrease with age, which is a major factor in whether we become ill or not in our later years.

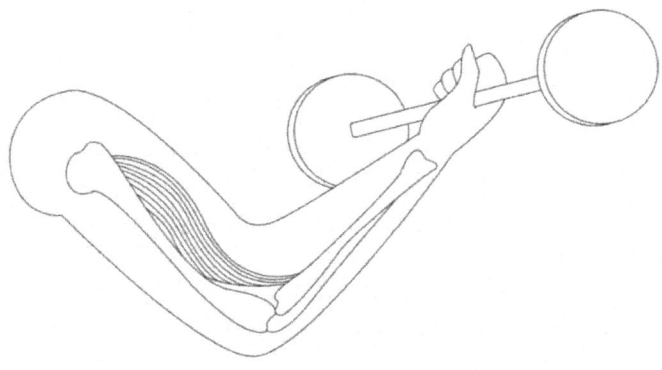

Regular resistance exercise keeps the body strong and muscle tissue vital throughout our life, which in turn will allow us to stay active, healthy, and independent for a lifetime. It's a necessary and positive stressor that's required to maintain strength and normal functioning of the skeletal system and metabolism.

The 5 Habits of Healthy People

The majority of people with type 2 diabetes, metabolic syndrome, chronic joint pain, and even many types of cancers can improve their conditions and symptoms significantly by doing consistent resistance exercise in combination with a diet that works for their particular body type and gastrointestinal (GI) system.

Today, resistance exercise is becoming more mainstream and accessible for a greater number of people. The gym attracts a certain crowd that prefers the shared experience of exercising together. But it's definitely not for everybody.

Personally, I never found the gym particularly appealing and preferred to exercise on my own at home or outside. I know many people also have the same feelings about the gym. Fortunately, resistance exercise isn't limited to a gym and includes any type of exercise that places a load (force) against your muscles. Some common types of resistance exercise include:

- Using body weight to do push-ups, planks, and squats
- Yoga and Pilates, which combine resistance exercise movements using body weight with stretching and flexibility work

Technology has also changed the health and fitness industry by making instructional fitness videos available for immediate streaming online. New fusion classes are also offered both online and in studios, blending different types of cardio and resistance exercises. The internet offers an avalanche of easily accessible health information. Health trackers and fitness gadgets also give us relatively easy ways to monitor and track our health and fitness.

The 5 Habits of Healthy People

All these factors have contributed to a growing collective awareness of how important resistance exercise is to living a long and healthy life.

Start with 15 Minutes

For someone just starting out with resistance exercise, start with 15 minutes a day. This will change over time as your conditioning and strength improve. The goal is to get to 30 minutes per day, every day, with a goal of doing 180 minutes per week.

Start with 15 minutes of resistance exercise and work up to a total of 30 minutes per day.

You can break up the 30-minutes-per-day goal into shorter sessions. For example, you can do two 15-minute sessions, three 10-minute sessions or one 30-minute session. It's up to you. What's important is that all of your sessions throughout the day total 30 minutes. That's the goal for consistent benefits.

The second edition of the *Physical Activity Guidelines for Americans*, released in 2018 by the Department of Health and Human Services, reports that 80 percent of adults are not meeting the minimum guidelines for both aerobic and muscle-strengthening exercise, while only about half meet the guidelines for aerobic physical activity. This lack of physical activity is linked to approximately $117 billion in annual health-care costs and about 10 percent of premature deaths.[7]

Most people benefit best by doing low-to-moderate resistance exercise every day, instead of doing a high-intensity version twice a week with rest days in between.

Their actual recommendation for resistance exercise says, "Adults should also do muscle-strengthening exercises of moderate or greater intensity that involves all major muscle groups on two or more days a week."

This recommendation is not only vague and unclear but also dated and less than ideal for most people. Why do I say this? One reason is that while it's true that lifting heavy weights intensely requires a rest period of a day or more in between exercise sessions, heavy weights are not what we are recommending for the average person.

To benefit from doing resistance exercise, most people don't need to do traditional bench presses with giant barbells and heavy weights, so they don't need long rest periods in between sessions. I personally do resistance exercise daily and from my experience believe that doing some every day is more beneficial and easier to maintain than a vague program of some resistance exercise of moderate to high intensity a couple of times a week. The habit of doing daily resistance exercise, when implemented over the long term, has the power to change the downward spiral that America's health has taken over the last 20 years.

Chronic Diseases and Their Relation to Muscle Mass

A healthy percentage of muscle is essential to physical well-being. After years of seeing patients, I have observed a definite pattern. As a person's muscle percentage decreases (usually after age 30), so does the person's metabolism and overall health. The metabolism is intimately connected to and depends on the body's skeletal muscle to power it and function optimally. Once a person's muscle starts to decrease below healthy levels, chronic health problems really start to kick in.

Holding on to your muscle throughout life is the closest thing to a "fountain of youth" you'll ever find.

Resistance exercise is also integral for proper blood sugar control, cardiovascular function, healthy blood pressure, injury prevention, and cancer risk reduction.

Diabetes

Type 2 diabetes is largely the result of lifestyle, with a minimal contribution from genetics. Having high blood pressure, high cholesterol, and high levels of sugar in your blood; being overweight or obese; smoking; being inactive; and consuming a diet rich in unnatural sweets and processed (synthetic or man-made) foods make it much more likely that a person will acquire diabetes.

Diabetes has reached alarming levels in the United States. In a 2015 study, the American Diabetes Association found that more than 30 million (over 9 percent of the adult population) had diabetes. Of the 30 million adults with diabetes, close to one-quarter, about 7.5 million, were undiagnosed. And another 84 million had prediabetes, a condition that if not corrected, often leads to type 2 diabetes within five years.[8]

This report and many others show that the problem is getting much worse compared to just 10 years ago. The total estimated cost for diagnosed diabetes in the United States in 2017 was $327 billion, making it one of the most expensive and damaging public health problems that we've seen in the modern era.[8] These numbers are surely higher if we include those who are currently undiagnosed.

Diabetes is insidious. It causes a variety of nonspecific symptoms such as fatigue; unexplained fluctuations in weight; changes in vision, eventually leading to vision loss; excessive thirst and urination; intraoral sores; nerve damage, leading to neuropathy (loss of sensation or chronic burning pain in the hands and feet); and chronic kidney disease, which eventually leads to kidney failure. Diabetes has been consistently one of the top 10 causes of death in the United States since the epidemic began 30–40 years ago.[9]

Diabetes Is Behavior Linked

Diabetes is largely a disease caused by what we eat and by our actions and inactions. The food we ingest is broken down into glucose, which is a form of sugar that our bodies use for energy production. Glucose is the main energy source for our bodies and is used directly (without the need for insulin) by certain tissues such as the brain, liver, and red blood cells under normal conditions.

The sugar (glucose) in food triggers the pancreas to release a hormone called insulin, which is required to drive sugar into muscle and fat cells. It does this by binding to the insulin receptors on muscle and fat cells, which opens up channels (transporters) in the cells to take up the sugar.

When the body has consistently high levels of sugar in the blood, the body will overproduce insulin. Over time, this makes the insulin receptors less sensitive to its effects (also called insulin insensitivity), so the blood sugar is no longer driven into the muscle and fat cells through the transporters that normally open up when binding with insulin.

One way to test for diabetes is to check fasting blood-sugar levels for several days in a row (at least three or more). The more data points we gather, the more confident we can be about where we lie on the spectrum, from normal blood-sugar levels to prediabetic blood-sugar levels to diabetes. Another important test to get is called the hemoglobin A1C. I advise you to have your doctor order a hemoglobin AIC test, which is a marker of blood-sugar levels over a longer period of time (weeks to months). An A1C test is also used to check how well people with diabetes are controlling their blood-sugar levels over time. The A1C test is the gold standard for determining ongoing blood-sugar levels and the effectiveness of treatment for diabetes.

New research is showing that resistance exercise has a greater effect on reducing A1C levels than aerobic exercise. One study in the *International Journal of Sports Medicine* showed that subjects who performed three months of moderate-intensity resistance exercise increased lean muscle mass significantly and showed a significant reduction in hemoglobin A1C levels. Aerobic exercise was also studied but did not show the same degree of long-term effects on lowering A1C levels.[10]

Research shows that resistance exercise has a greater effect on reducing excessive blood sugar levels over the long term.

Resistance exercise has also been shown to improve insulin sensitivity (reverse diabetes) by increasing insulin sensitivity by 23 percent in a study published in *Hormone and Metabolic Research* whereas no change in insulin sensitivity occurred in the aerobic exercise test group. The study's authors recommended including resistance exercise in prevention programs for individuals at risk of developing diabetes.[11]

A study published in the *Journal of Clinical Endocrinology and Metabolism* showed that both aerobic and resistance exercise improved the body's ability to absorb glucose more than either aerobic exercise alone or resistance exercise alone. For individuals with obesity, arthritis, nerve pain, or other physical disabilities, who find aerobic exercise such as walking, biking, or running uncomfortable or even painful, regular low-impact resistance exercise is a must.[12]

Along with activity levels, monitor your intake of carbohydrates, specifically refined (artificial and concentrated) carbohydrates, to help prevent the onset of insulin resistance, diabetes, and other diseases like atherosclerosis that are related to chronically high blood-sugar levels. We will discuss how to test your blood-sugar levels at home in the chapter on Keystone Health Measurements (Habit #5).

Cardiovascular Disease

It is now known that resistance exercise is an essential component for reducing risk factors of cardiovascular or heart disease, which is the leading cause of death each year in the United States.[13] A study in the *Lancet* found that having more muscular strength is inversely associated with all-cause mortality, including heart attacks and strokes.[14]

About half of all Americans have at least one risk factor for heart disease, including high blood pressure, elevated cholesterol, obesity, or tobacco use. In addition, inactivity, a poor diet, and consuming more than a moderate amount of alcohol on a regular basis will also increase your risk.

Research shows that both aerobic exercise and resistance exercise produce beneficial effects on blood vessels, and both types of exercise are equally important for optimal heart health. Resistance exercise has been shown to increase blood flow to surrounding tissues. Aerobic exercise has been shown to increase arterial elasticity, which is an artery's ability to expand and contract smoothly. Because of its ability to increase blood flow while being able to lower the heart rate, resistance exercise is also recommended for heart patients in cardiac rehabilitation programs.[15,16]

Today, one in three US adults (about 85 million people) has high blood pressure.[17] Resistance exercise has been shown to lower high blood pressure for longer periods following exercise than aerobic exercise.[18] Researchers think this may be due to the increased blood flow to more tissues as well as the improved blood flow that results from the muscle contraction that comes with resistance exercise. Resistance exercise has also been found to reduce systolic blood pressure more than aerobic exercise when the two were compared.[19]

Research published in *Sports Medicine* demonstrated that resistance exercise has a strong association with improved total cholesterol levels and the levels of lipids (bad fats) in the blood. Resistance exercise has also been shown to reduce the levels of low-density lipoproteins or LDL, also known as bad cholesterol, while increasing the levels of good high-density lipoproteins or HDL cholesterol. This is certainly better than taking a cholesterol-lowering drug such as a statin for life.[20]

*Resistance exercise helps to lower the bad LDL
cholesterol and increase the good HDL.*

Stroke patients also benefit from resistance exercise. It helps them to regain muscular strength and mobility and decrease contractures (shortening and wasting of muscles, tendons, and ligaments). This is extremely important, as contractures can cause rigid joints and muscular imbalances that impede a person's ability to live independently following a stroke.[21]

The American Heart Association recommends resistance exercise at least two days a week in addition to 30 minutes per day of aerobic exercise. Again, this recommendation is dated and vague and not based on any real science or data. I recommend setting a goal of doing 30 minutes a day of low- to moderate-intensity resistance exercise every day that is timed rather than based on sets and reps (see chapter on the Gravity Ball Method™).

Cancer

Resistance exercise also improves the lives of patients undergoing treatment for cancer. The American Cancer Society refers to at least 20 different studies that demonstrate physically active cancer survivors have a lower risk of cancer returning and longer life expectancy than inactive cancer survivors. Resistance exercise has been shown to increase total body muscle and reduce the side effects of cancer treatment.[22]

Although researchers do not know exactly how resistance exercise helps reduce the effects of cancer and cancer treatments, they're sure that including it as part of a cancer treatment program has immense benefits. It is now clear that muscle activation during exercise helps upregulate the immune system, activating various immune cells that can target and destroy cancer cells. The increased blood flow also helps carry the chemotherapy drugs to the cancer sites for more effective actions.

New research out of Australia shows incredible benefits when new cancer patients start targeted exercise programs that include both aerobic and resistance exercise. Patients with different types of cancer receive tailored exercise programs directly after receiving their chemotherapy treatments. Low-impact resistance exercise helps maintain strength and energy levels, which are significantly reduced during treatment. Exercises that involved jumping paired with resistance exercise reduced high-degree bone loss associated with large drops in testosterone after treatment for prostate cancer.[23]

Resistance exercise helps cancer patients maintain strength and energy levels, which can suffer during treatment.

The American Cancer Society recommends 150 minutes of aerobic exercise and two days a week of strengthening exercise for those recovering from or who are living with a stable condition. It's important for cancer patients or survivors to work with their physicians and exercise specialists to determine the specific limitations they are facing in order to help them determine which type of exercise is best for them. This is best done with the help of a physical therapist and an experienced exercise trainer who is familiar with working with people who have been through cancer treatment.

Injury Risk

Resistance exercise not only increases muscle size and strength but also promotes growth and increases in strength of ligaments and tendons, which are the tissues that connect bones and muscles to joints. This results in stronger joints and increases in bone density, which reduces the likelihood of breaking or fracturing bones. These are critical factors that make the body stronger and much more resistant to injuries.

I see overuse injuries regularly in my practice. Some of the most common overuse injuries include carpal tunnel syndrome (wrist tendonitis), tennis elbow (inflammation to the elbow tendons), shoulder problems such as rotator cuff problems, runner's knee (misalignment of the knee cap), Achilles tendonitis, and shin splints (microfractures in the shin bone).

Overuse injuries happen over time through repetitive movements and actions that injure the bones, muscles, tendons, or ligaments. Practicing regular resistance exercise with good form and technique will significantly reduce your chances of developing these types of overuse injuries.

Chronic Pain

Acute pain signals are generated by the nervous system when we injure ourselves. These signals prevent further injury by forcing us to remove ourselves from any situation that will cause more pain. Chronic pain is a type of pain that may get better or worse over time but never really goes away. This type of pain continues for weeks, months, or years, resulting in both physical and mental suffering.

According to the National Institutes of Health (NIH), 11.2 percent of Americans (or about 25 million people) have experienced or continue to experience some form of chronic pain each day.[24] It can be the result of genetics, trauma, infection, muscle atrophy (muscle loss), or a previous injury. Chronic pain can also stem from conditions such as fibromyalgia, rheumatoid arthritis, osteoarthritis, chronic fatigue syndrome, and endometriosis.

Treating chronic pain differs from treating acute pain that may happen from a sprained ankle or a torn muscle, which will typically heal relatively quickly with rest and over-the-counter pain medication. Chronic pain is more complex and often involves multiple factors such as one's state of physical and metabolic health and emotional and psychological states. For this reason, there is no general treatment that can be used for everybody.

Each person requires a personalized treatment that can only be determined over time and with continuous observation and adjusting of the treatment based on the person's symptoms and response to the treatment. Oftentimes, alternative treatments can offer significant relief in symptoms and improve well-being. It is no secret that prescription narcotic painkillers have terrible side effects and are extremely addictive. But did you know that they can also delay healing and prolong or worsen many disease states? [25]

Many people with chronic pain lose the ability to work and enjoy life. This type of pain can lead to depression, a reduced ability to concentrate, and excessive fatigue, making even the simplest tasks overwhelming.

Chronic pain can have both neurological and physical components. Research has shown that people in chronic pain may have reduced neuroplasticity, affecting the ability of the brain to adapt to new changes and experiences. A constant pain signal can also cause abnormal neural wiring, which can make you hypersensitive to pain and keep you in a constant state of stress.[26]

Exercise has been shown to improve the brain's neuroplasticity by increasing blood flow, oxygen, and vital growth factors to the brain. Yoga, Pilates, or tai chi are forms of resistance exercise that improve physical function, enhance quality of life, and reduce pain in those who have chronic pain from various causes.[27]

Resistance exercise helps improve chronic pain symptoms by increasing blood flow and healing processes within the brain and body and also by strengthening muscles of joints for those with joint pain due to muscle loss.

Resistance exercise is also the best way to reduce pain and improve function in people who suffer from chronic lower back pain, knee osteoarthritis, and chronic tendon problems (tendinopathies) of various joints. The muscles that stabilize our joints are also responsible for protecting the bones of the joints by acting as shock absorbers so that minimal stress and contact of the bones at the joint takes place. Building up the muscle groups that support the joints is the best way to prevent injury and to reduce chronic pain in those with chronic joint pains.

Mental Health

Over the years I've seen many people with depression, anxiety, schizophrenia, bipolar disorder, posttraumatic stress disorder (PTSD), or some combination of mental-health issues. Mental illness can stem from a variety of factors, including genetic predispositions, upbringing, events that happen in life and lifestyle choices. Following patients over the years, I've noticed that those who are able to optimize their lifestyles for healthy living improve their mental health to a much higher degree without the need for medications than those who simply rely on taking antidepressant medications.

The 5 Habits of Healthy People

*Those who can optimize their lifestyles for
healthy living will often become more mentally
healthy without the need for medications.*

It's believed that exercise helps regulate hormonal production and build new neural pathways (nerve connections) through increased neurotransmitters that stimulate nerve cell growth in patients diagnosed with depression, according to research published in *Journal of Lifestyle Medicine*, although we don't know exactly how.[28] A study in *Frontiers in Psychology* also showed that low- to moderate-intensity resistance exercise reduces anxiety.[29]

Aging

Older adults tend to lose muscle, have weaker bones, gain weight due to increased accumulation of body fat, and have a significantly increased decline in cognition. This doesn't have to be the case.

I believe that this trend has become accepted by society as normal, which is why you often hear the sayings, "It sucks to get old" or "That's what happens when you get old." I do not believe that we are destined to disease with age. It's the cumulative effects of inactivity over a lifetime that's the culprit.

Our senior years can be greatly enhanced with a program of consistent resistance exercise. The benefits are numerous and include improved muscle and bone health, preservation of metabolic health, and protection against cognitive decline in conditions such as Alzheimer's and dementia. A 2016 study in *Journal of American Geriatrics* on men and women aged 55 through 86 with mild cognitive impairment found that when they performed weight-based exercises twice weekly for six months, they significantly improved their scores on various cognitive tests.[30]

Maintaining your muscle mass becomes increasingly important as you get older. Think of your muscle as the currency of your "life force or vitality" account. It's the most important thing to hold onto for the rest of your life. Muscle strength is necessary for a normal and healthy metabolism. It will keep you leaner and fitter now and in the future. All you have to do is incorporate resistance exercise into your daily routine. It just takes 30 minutes a day.

We're not doomed to deteriorate as we age.
Inactivity is the culprit. Think of your muscle as the
currency of your "life savings" account.

You can build muscle at any age to maintain your health now and in later years. A study in *Preventive Medicine* found an incredible 46 percent reduction in premature all-cause mortality in adults who did the recommended amount of resistance exercise, compared with those who did not.[31]

The benefits of resistance exercise span a lifetime, from improving high blood pressure and increasing insulin sensitivity to reducing injury risk and increasing the odds of surviving against cancer. The array of benefits that it provides is truly amazing.

My mission is to make resistance exercise as widely popular and as widely practiced as cardio-based exercise is now. And you're never too old to start.

The 5 Habits of Healthy People

Current Recommendations versus Our Recommendations

The American College of Sports Medicine recommends that healthy adults perform a minimum of two nonconsecutive days of resistance exercise each week. I don't agree with this recommendation. This is not enough to make it a habit, which is what our goal is.

I recommend that most healthy adults work their way up to doing 30 minutes per day: a 30-minute session, two 15-minute, or three 10-minute sessions, it's up to you as long as you total 30 minutes at the end of the day. Adults with various chronic conditions will likely need a modified version of this daily plan.

I recommend most healthy adults perform 30 minutes of daily resistance exercise, this can be broken up into several sessions depending on your schedule.

Now as with anything, there's a right way and a wrong way to do resistance exercise. Weights that are too heavy or exercises that are done with improper form can cause serious injury. Do only essential joint movements and limit nonessential repetitions and jerky movements to preserve joint function, promote proper body mechanics, and heighten your awareness of muscular and joint imbalances.

This is why I created the Gravity Ball Method™. I saw that people (myself included) needed a better and more accessible way to do safe, effective, and consistent daily resistance exercise. The Gravity Ball Method utilizes static and non-static movements with a new weighted-exercise device called the Gravity Ball™ to improve balance, symmetry between both halves of the body, flexibility, mobility, and strength; more on this later.

Chapter 2

Habit #2: Daily Movement and Steps

Cardiovascular (aerobic) exercise (a.k.a. "cardio") is exercise that gets the heart rate up and keeps it up for some period of time or distance. Cardio exercise stimulates circulation, blood flow, and oxygen delivery, and it strengthens your heart. Some common examples of cardio exercise include running, swimming, and bicycling.

Although cardio is now "a thing," it hasn't always been popular. The connection of exercise to health didn't take hold in America until the 1950s. Reports from World War I had shown that most of the draftees were unfit for combat. So, the government passed laws that required that school physical-education programs improve the quality of their curriculum to improve the fitness of the students. The Great Depression derailed that focus while everyone was trying to figure out how to survive the hard times.

During World War II, nearly half of all draftees again were found unfit for combat and were relegated to noncombat positions. In 1950s and 1960s, the government backed new fitness initiatives to lift the spirits and the health of demoralized Americans. In 1954, the

American College of Sports Medicine was created. Then, in 1956, the President's Council on Youth Fitness was created to encourage greater levels of fitness among young people. (President Kennedy later changed the name to The President's Council on Physical Fitness in 1963 to include all Americans.)[32]

A Nation of Couch Potatoes

The 1950's saw America come into its own. The country was prospering, and most Americans now enjoyed the comforts of suburban living, including one of America's favorite pastimes: watching television. Great numbers of "couch potatoes" became unhealthy and overweight as people watched more and more television, became less active, and started eating more processed foods. Thus, the modern diabetes epidemic that is now on everybody's radar screen was born.

Jack LaLanne, one of America's favorite health pioneers, vowed to combat this trend by utilizing television to get his message out about health. The Jack LaLanne Show ran from 1951 until 1985. LaLanne was a bodybuilder, an author, and a founding father of fitness. He taught his viewers how to do both aerobic and strength-training exercise at home. He had transformed his own life through food and exercise and believed that the nation's health was dependent on the health of each individual American. He changed the lives of thousands of Americans and paved the way for other health and fitness advocates.

Around this same time, Dr. Thomas K. Cureton, a professor at the University of Illinois known as "the father of physical fitness," was researching the mechanisms of exercise to understand the benefits of exercise scientifically. His recommendations included exercising for six days a week, a demand that many questioned at the time. Dr.

Cureton helped Americans see exercise as a positive force that would add years to their lives.[33]

Dr. Jeremy N. Morris, a British epidemiologist had also begun his studies on the heart-attack rates for double-decker bus drivers and conductors in London. His study began the research field of aerobic activity and heart health. He found that the conductors (who climbed stairs throughout their shift) had less than half the heart-attack rates as the sedentary drivers.[34]

By the 1960s, aerobic exercise was growing in popularity. In 1968, the term "aerobics" was coined by Dr. Kenneth H. Cooper, who authored the internationally best-selling book *Aerobics. The Jogger's Manual,* published in 1963, was a 250-word pamphlet that popularized cardio-based exercise. The manual was published by University of Oregon track and field coach Bill Bowerman and the future cofounder of Nike, Phil Knight, who developed the original Nike running shoes. *The Jogger's Manual* inspired many to begin running at a time when it wasn't commonplace.[35]

The 1970s and 1980s ushered in Jazzercise, the jazz-inspired aerobic and strength full-body fitness program, and the flamboyant and lovable Richard Simmons, who popularized dance aerobics that offered high-energy dance movements for weight loss. In the 1990s, step classes and Billy Blank's Tae Bo popularized kickboxing and step aerobics, which gained further support for the cardio movement.[36]

Today, aerobic exercise is recognized as essential to staying healthy and is practiced by people of all ages. But many people still don't do it, at least, not regularly.

As discussed in Habit #1, resistance exercise builds and maintains muscle mass, which is important for many vital processes in our body.

Aerobic exercise, on the other hand, is focused on improving the circulatory and respiratory systems.

These systems provide oxygen delivery as well as other vital nutrients to our tissues and remove waste from the body, so the body can continue to function optimally. The cardiorespiratory system is also crucial for maintaining proper fluid balance and blood pressure.

Guidelines from the CDC recommend that adults do at least 2.5 hours of moderate-intensity aerobic activity weekly, or 75 minutes of vigorous activity a week.

It's easy to take 10,000 steps a day because you already do some walking. An extra flight of stairs, or a more distant parking space can add steps to your count painlessly.

Step It Up!

Rather than having to take up running, swimming, biking or other cardio-based sport, a daily step count is a good way to measure and keep track of your daily movement (cardio activity). It's easy to measure with today's cell phones and activity trackers.

If you don't walk much or have been sedentary for some time, a good goal to start with is anywhere from 6,000 to 8,000 steps a day and work up to a goal of averaging 10,000 steps, (or approximately five miles) every day. That's about twice the current average. (If you need a rule of thumb, think of every mile equaling about 2,000 steps.)

Do you think 10,000 steps sounds like a lot? You'd be surprised at how easily your steps mount up when you take an extra flight of stairs or park a little farther from your building or walk down the hall to talk to a colleague instead of calling or emailing.

10,000 step count is about having a clear goal
for your activity each day

The 10,000-step daily goal is more about having a clear goal to aim for each day. It's very simple: at the end of the day, did you reach 10,000 steps? Yes or no. Over time (over months and years), you will learn how often you're hitting your daily goal. Using a step-tracking method, you'll be able to develop habits that last a lifetime.

Chapter 3

Habit #3: 80/20 Eating

The 80/20 eating plan favors healthy eating but also allows you to include foods that you like but are not considered healthy, like fast or processed food.

The concept of the 80/20 ratio is simple: 80 percent of the foods and meals you eat, ideally, come from foods that are wholesome, unprocessed or minimally processed, and natural occurring. The other 20 percent of meals and foods consumed can be fast foods, processed foods, or anything in between.

For example, if you eat three meals per day every day, then in seven days, you'll eat 21 meals. Of those 21 meals, 80 percent (or 17) of them are ideally meals that are made up of whole or unprocessed foods. This leaves four meals per week that can be of any food types you wish.

We can't list all of the many wholesome and healthy foods, but we can boil down the basic categories of foods that are universally unhealthy. Try to keep these unhealthy foods to about 20 percent of your total food intake.

The 5 Habits of Healthy People

Anything with artificial fats, sugars, colors or preservatives is unhealthy.

In general, unhealthy foods contain one or more of the following: artificial fats (trans fats and hydrogenated fats), artificial sugars, artificial colors, and artificial preservatives. The more of these four things a food contains, in general, the worse it is for your health. That makes it simple.

The goal is for 80 percent of your meals to be from natural and whole foods that contain as few of these four ingredients as possible. The healthiest foods have none of them.

For example, diet soda sounds innocuous. How could it be harmful if it has no calories? Here's the problem: it still contains artificial sugars, artificial colors, and artificial preservatives. It has three of the four "unhealthy food" criteria, so it shouldn't be included in more than 20 percent of your meals each week.

Why Not Diet?

Diets are almost always short-term thinking. They're not about changing behavior but rather stress willpower to resist certain foods for a short and usually unspecified period of time. Not having clear goals that end bad habits and create good habits and relying on willpower to avoid certain foods is not a healthy way to live and is not sustainable for long-term change.

Most diets are a one-size-fits-all, restrictive approach to choosing foods that apply the same rules to everyone. They have us avoiding entire food groups and living with restrictions of total calories or of certain food groups. This is not sustainable or necessary.

The Dangers of Restrictive and Extreme Weight-Loss Diets

Restrictive diets can leave out vital macro and micronutrients (vitamins and minerals) and other components of a healthy diet, such as fiber, which most people are deficient in. Blanket food restrictions are counterproductive unless they're due to a specific medical condition such as Crohn's disease, inflammatory bowel disease, or celiac disease, in which case a restrictive diet is often medically prescribed and beneficial.

Dieting for extreme weight loss is also dangerous. It can negatively affect your metabolism and your immune system, altering your body's ability to maintain normal organ function and fight off illness. When you suddenly and drastically reduce your calorie intake, this signals your body that it's in danger, and it will switch to a starvation (stress and inflammation) mode, which shocks the metabolism, causing it to shut down energy burning to an absolute minimum.

The result is that your baseline metabolic rate (the number of calories your body burns at rest) drops significantly, which means your body is using fewer calories per day. This is often the reason that people who are on very low-calorie diets can paradoxically gain weight or find it difficult to lose weight. Besides an impaired metabolism, significant muscle breakdown and muscle loss can result, as well as malnutrition, and nervous system dysfunction (poor memory, inability to concentrate, tingling, or numb hands and feet).

Our food choices shouldn't eliminate certain food groups or make large reductions in calories (although smaller restrictions of calories have a role for long-term weight loss). A good eating plan focuses on increasing the intake of beneficial nutrients and fiber that the body needs and taking in just enough calories to meet daily requirements.

A good food plan doesn't eliminate certain foods or make drastic reductions in calories but focuses on choosing good foods a majority of the time.

The beauty of the 80/20 system is its flexibility. It allows you to live a normal life. You might decide to use the 20 percent when having a meal out with friends or family or when you're on the go. This 80/20 approach to eating is a long-term approach, unlike restrictive diets.

The 80/20 approach allows us to enjoy any foods we chose to while still making healthy choices a good majority of the time. This approach to eating is sustainable, easy to understand, and easy to follow.

Examples of Meals in the 80 Percent

Breakfast: Cage-free and antibiotic-free omelet cooked with ghee (clarified butter) and filled with mushrooms, tomatoes, and spinach, plus black coffee;

Lunch: A hearty salad with nuts, raw vegetables, cage-free and antibiotic-free (organic) chicken, salmon, or turkey with avocado and a vinaigrette dressing;

Snack: Organic apple or other fruit and nuts, almond butter, tea;

Dinner: salmon or grass-fed beef (organic) with a side of roasted vegetables and a small side salad; and

Desert: Dark chocolate with some fresh blueberries, raspberries, or blackberries.

The 5 Habits of Healthy People

Choosing "Quality" Food

Consuming low-quality fuel (food) or not enough fuel is just like putting low-quality fuel in your car, which would cause it to run poorly and sputter. Our physical and mental health will sputter and be impaired when we put low-quality food in our bodies.

To function optimally, we need a consistent supply of several high-quality nutrients. The three major macronutrients include protein,

WHOLE FOODS
FOOD GROUP BREAKDOWN PER DAY

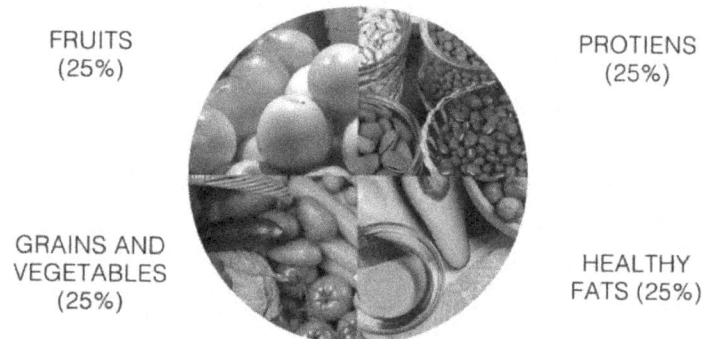

FRUITS
(25%)

PROTIENS
(25%)

GRAINS AND
VEGETABLES
(25%)

HEALTHY
FATS (25%)

carbohydrates, and fats. Also essential are vitamins, minerals, and adequate water intake.

So how much do you need from each group? One-quarter of your daily foods should come from each of the following four food groups: proteins (both plant and animal if you eat animal products), vegetables, fruits, and healthy fats.

Now, let's look more closely at these food groups.

The 5 Habits of Healthy People

Proteins

Proteins are the building blocks of the body. Having enough high-quality protein is essential for optimum health.

Why?

Our bodies rely on protein to grow new tissue and repair old and damaged tissue. It's also needed to produce essential hormones and enzymes that maintain a healthy metabolism and immune system and to keep the body's organs functioning properly.

The Recommended Dietary Allowance (RDA) is the minimum amount of protein recommended to maintain a healthy amount of muscle. As I write this book, the current RDA for protein is 0.8 grams of protein per kilogram of body weight in a 24-hour period.

A kilogram is 2.2 pounds. To gauge your weight in kilograms, divide by 2.2. Here's the conversion for a 130-pound person:

130lbs divided by 2.2 = 59 kg × 0.8 gram/kg (RDA) = 47 grams of protein. A 130-pound adult should be taking in about 50 grams of protein per day.

All protein is not created equal. Choose high-quality sources that offer a combo of the nine essential amino acids.

This "rule of thumb" is good enough for most people. We recommend eating a minimum of 40 grams of protein per day, depending on your gender, your activity level, and your specific body type. Most healthy and active people should be consuming between 50 and 100 grams of protein per day. If you're very active and do a lot of physical work or exercise, the amount of protein you take in each day will be more than someone of the same weight and gender who is less active.

Remember, all protein is not created equal. Choose high-quality sources of proteins that offer a combination of the nine essential amino acids.

Twenty different amino acids make up all the proteins in our food and in our body. Nine of these are considered essential amino acids. The body cannot convert any of the 11 nonessential amino acids into the nine essential amino acids, and therefore, they must be taken in through diet.

The foods in the following list are the most common sources of essential amino acids:

- Meat, eggs, soy, black beans, quinoa, and pumpkin seeds
- Fish, poultry, nuts, seeds, and whole grains
- Cottage cheese and wheat germ
- Soy, cheese, peanuts, mushrooms, whole grains, and vegetables
- Dairy, beans, and legumes
- Chicken and turkey

These are just a few examples of foods that are rich in essential amino acids. All foods that contain protein, whether plant based or animal based, will contain some essential amino acids.[37]

Oftentimes your diet can be improved significantly simply by increasing the quality of the proteins you consume. This can be done in part by reducing the intake of non-nutritious foods and substituting them with quality sources of protein.

The 5 Habits of Healthy People

Examples of quality protein sources include: organic grass-fed beef (portion size of 2–4 oz, (about the size of an iPhone or deck of cards, depending on cut and thickness), free-range and antibiotic-free poultry, cage-free eggs, wild-caught fish (salmon, cod, trout, sardines, mackerel), egg-white protein powder, black beans, brown rice, and quinoa. Consuming animal organ meats (liver, kidney, heart) is also a good way to increase essential nutrients like the fat-soluble vitamins A, D, E, and K while getting quality protein. Aim to obtain around 25 percent of your daily caloric intake from high-quality protein sources.

Carbohydrates: Your Body's Main Fuel

Carbohydrates provide the body with its main source of fuel to perform its essential functions throughout the day. There are two classes of carbohydrates: simple and complex. Simple carbohydrates consist of one or two sugar molecules (see image below) and include fruits, root vegetables, natural sugars such as honey and maple syrup, and naturally occurring sugars in dairy products. These simple sugar molecules are absorbed faster into the bloodstream, as they don't need to be broken down as much by the GI tract. They also lack the non-digestible fibers found in complex carbohydrates that slow down the digestion of the complex forms of sugars.

SIMPLE SUGARS   COMPLEX SUGARS

The 5 Habits of Healthy People

Carbs have been getting a bad rap. Complex carbs contain fiber and are metabolized more slowly than simple carbs, keeping hunger at bay for longer.

Complex carbohydrates have longer chains of sugar molecules and, as a result of these chains, contain higher amounts of fiber, which means these sugars are broken down more slowly and released into the bloodstream at a much slower and steadier rate. This provides a steady and consistent amount of blood sugar over time and avoids rapid spikes and crashes in blood-sugar levels that come with consuming too many simple sugars. Some sources of complex carbohydrates include brown rice, grains, steel-cut oats (oatmeal), quinoa, beans, and lentils. High-fiber carbohydrates also tend to have more nutrients because they're likely to be whole foods that have not been processed.

Our brains utilize sugar as their main source of fuel and are powered mainly from the simple sugar glucose that passes easily through the blood-brain barrier. This is one of the main reasons that maintaining proper blood-sugar levels is so important.

Our brains depend on it.

Your brain depends on maintaining proper blood sugar levels.

Aim to obtain 50 percent of your daily foods from fruits, vegetables, and grains, which should include mostly complex carbohydrates contained in foods such as whole grain-sprouted breads;

brown rice; quinoa; vegetables such as broccoli, asparagus, spinach, and kale; and fruits such as apples and berries (of all types).

Fats for Survival

Fats are an important part of a healthy body, brain, and nervous system, yet there's still a lot of confusion about which fats are good and which ones are bad.

Fats cushion our joints and protect our organs. Fat helps insulate us from the cold and provides the body with a reservoir to absorb and store fat-soluble vitamins and other nutrients that are essential for a healthy nervous system.

There are four types of fats: saturated, monounsaturated, polyunsaturated, and trans fats. As a general rule of thumb, saturated fats are usually solid at room temperature. Think butter, coconut oil, and most animal fats. Unsaturated fats are usually liquid at room temperature and are found in vegetable and fruit oils such olive oil, grapeseed oil, and avocado oil.

Ignore the controversy linking saturated fats to heart disease. It's a time-tested ploy by the food industries, and saturated fats eaten in moderation are fine. Saturated fats such as fats from animal meat, dairy, and butter also get a bad rap. However, having some animal-based saturated fats from organic sources is fine if you just apply the 80/20 principle. This means that approximately 20 percent of the total amount of fats you consume daily can be of the saturated type. The other 80 percent ideally will be from monounsaturated and polyunsaturated fats.

Remember that saturated fats have been an important source of energy throughout history. Maasai warriors have survived on three-to-five liters of whole milk each day and high amounts of fatty meat when available as well as animal blood. Their blood pressure was found to be 50 percent lower than the average American's blood pressure, and it didn't rise with age (something we increasingly expect in aging Americans.) They also had no evidence of heart disease even in the older men who have lower activity levels.[38]

Synthetic Fats: Just Say No

We do recommend that you avoid fats that have been processed and synthetically made. These types of fats can react with other molecules or cells in your body and cause inflammation and cell damage. Fortunately, the FDA has banned the use of trans fats by food manufactures. This ban went into effect on June 18, 2018; products manufactured before this date can still be distributed until January 2020, or in some cases 2021.[39]

In general, processed foods such as crackers, cookies, cakes, frozen pies, other baked goods, snack foods (such as microwave popcorn), frozen pizza, vegetable shortenings, some stick margarines, coffee creamers, refrigerated dough products (such as biscuits and cinnamon rolls), and ready-to-use frostings are typical foods that contain the most amount of trans fats (which are also called partially hydrogenated fats).

We recommend obtaining the vast majority of your fats from the natural, unsaturated plant-based fats such as avocado oil, olive oil, nuts, seeds, nut butters, coconut oil, and eggs as well as some fatty fish such as sardines and salmon. Also, include some saturated fats from high-quality animal sources, if you eat meat. Keep your fat consumption to about 25 percent of your daily calorie intake.

Keep your fat consumption to about 25 percent of your daily calorie intake.

The 5 Habits of Healthy People

Lifestyle plays a huge role in how the nutrition from our food is processed by our bodies, and sometimes things will get to us. It's not just the foods we eat. Our stress levels, the amount of sleep we get, our sense of knowing how we feel after eating certain foods, and the types of activities we take part in all affect our nutritional state.

Take a good look at your lifestyle. Are you staying in control of your stress levels, sleep levels, and the foods you eat? Heightened awareness will help you make healthy choices more consistently.

With the 80/20 principle, we've simplified eating, so you don't have to think so much about each meal, reducing stress. It makes eating healthily more sustainable than extreme diets, which eventually deplete even the strongest willpower. As a general guideline, 80 percent of your meals should include high-quality whole foods that provide high amounts of nutrients. Over time, choosing which foods to eat will become much easier and more intuitive.

Heightened awareness of your lifestyle – stress levels, quality and quantity of sleep and food quality – will help you make more consistent health decisions.

A Few More Recommendations

Organic Foods

Organic foods are foods grown without synthetic fertilizers, herbicides, or pesticides. Organic farms only use natural methods for fertilizing, pest control, and crop rotation, practices that are less harmful to the environment. Organic grass-fed livestock isn't fed growth hormones or given antibiotics. Organic foods also do not contain genetically modified organisms (GMOs).

Nonorganically grown produce often contains pesticides that have been linked to the development of chronic conditions such as diabetes and cancer, neurodegenerative diseases such as Alzheimer's disease, dementia, and Parkinson's disease, and developmental delays in children.[40]

We advise buying organic foods whenever possible and whenever you can afford it, not only for the improved taste but for the increase in nutrition and the reduction in exposure to unnecessary chemicals and pesticides. We recommend referring to the Dirty Dozen™ and the Clean 15™ lists of foods with the lowest and highest amount of pesticides to accordingly choose which items to buy organically. The lists are updated annually by the Environmental Working Group (EWG).[41]

Coffee

There are many health benefits associated with drinking moderate amounts of coffee. For one thing, it's rich in antioxidants. A study in *Annals of Internal Medicine* found coffee consumption to be associated with lower all-cause mortality from a variety of diseases.[42]

Coffee has also been shown to protect against liver disease and various cancers and to reduce the symptoms of depression.[43]

Caffeine can cause a minor increase in blood pressure and heart rate, so this is something to be aware of if you have a heart condition or high blood pressure. However, the effects of raising the blood pressure and heart rate are usually brief and decrease over time. Genes determine how each of us processes and metabolizes caffeine, so listen to your body, and adjust your intake up or down to maximize benefits and minimize negative effects.[44]

Overall, the benefits of drinking coffee make it well worth considering as part of your daily beverage intake.

Coffee is rich in antioxidants and protects against liver disease and various cancers, and reduces symptoms of depression.

Alcohol

Alcohols such as wines, ciders, and beers can provide antioxidants and B vitamins and aid in digestion. Beer and wine (and coffee) have been shown to lower the risks of kidney stones and moderate alcohol consumption (one glass of wine at dinner) may even help boost the immune system.[45,46]

While a small amount of wine may be beneficial, we do not recommend drinking alcohol, except on occasion such as on a holiday or at a significant celebration.

Dairy

We recommend keeping cow's milk and dairy products made from cow's milk to a minimum. Dairy milk (from cows) does contain some beneficial nutrients. However, because the proteins and sugar in cow's milk are not easily digested by most people, milk can cause problems with digestion and gut inflammation (leaky gut), leading to gas, bloating, diarrhea, and other negative secondary effects such as allergic and immune reactions that increase total body inflammation.

Plant-based milks like almond, coconut or soy milk are easier to digest than cow's milk.

We suggest replacing cow's milk and dairy with nut-based milk such as almond, coconut, or soy milk. These plant-based milks are much easier to digest and will not cause the inflammation, bloating, and diarrhea that often happen with dairy products, which can lead to poor absorption of nutrients in the GI tract.

Artificial Sweeteners

Artificial sweeteners are highly processed synthetic sugar substitutes that are designed to replace sucrose or table sugar. They are typically much higher in sweetness than regular sugar, as the molecules (chemicals) in most of them bind to taste buds much more strongly than do the molecules of sugar in table sugar. Saccharin is 300 times sweeter than table sugar; aspartame is 200 times sweeter.

Each artificial sweetener tastes different because of their varying molecular shape, which affects how they bind to taste receptors. They're popular in sugar-free or diet products, prepared low-calorie desserts, and sweets. One teaspoon of table sugar has about 16 calories, and one can of sweetened cola with 10 teaspoons of added sugar has about 160 calories, which, when replaced with an artificial sweetener, will have zero calories or very few calories.

Because they do not contain any calories and are not able to be metabolized by our bodies, they cannot raise our blood-sugar levels. However, they can potentially cause us to overeat, as our brain stops associating sweetness with calories and fullness, causing us to have more servings.

We don't metabolize artificial sweeteners so they don't raise our blood sugar. It's deceptive. The truth is, they can do more harm than good.

We recommend not using artificial sweeteners or products that contain them. Overall, it's good practice to limit the portion and frequency of sugar-sweetened foods you eat, and when you do eat them, have them for an occasional indulgence or celebration. If you're going to use an artificial sweetener, we suggest using Stevia, as it is from a plant.

Supplements

We do recommend taking high-quality supplements when there is likely a deficiency in your diet. In my experience, many people are deficient in vitamins A, D, E, K, some of the B vitamins (thiamin, folate), calcium, and magnesium. Women also tend to be low in iron, especially those who have heavy and prolonged menstrual cycles and those who are vegetarians or vegans. We recommend getting your blood tested with an online service like WellnessFX.com, or go through your doctor in order to see if you have any deficiencies before beginning with specific supplements.

Find out more about supplements at labdoor.com. I personally use supplements from Thorne and Kion.

The 5 Habits of Healthy People

Water

Water makes up close to 60 percent of our total body composition. It is vital to regulating pH balance and body temperature, lubricating the joints, and regulating and eliminating waste and excess toxins.

We've all heard the recommendation that we drink at least eight glasses of water per day. However, water intake should be based on your activity levels and environmental conditions. If you're more active, are sweating more, and are in a hot and humid environment, you will need to consume more water throughout the day to avoid becoming dehydrated and the negative effects that happen with dehydration. As a general rule, I advise the people I work with to drink enough water and other beverages throughout the day so that their urine remains clear to light yellow in color.

Chapter 4

Habit #4: Sound Sleep

In an ideal world, to optimize our health and well-being, we'd spend about one-third of our lives asleep. But the busier we get, the more tempting it becomes to sacrifice an hour of sleep here or two hours there in order to spend time with family, send those last emails, or catch up on a show we've been missing.

Personally, sleep deprivation and I have become close over the years, from the many all-nighters I pulled in medical school to the 24-hour, 36-hour, and 48-hour shifts I spent on call during residency training and during my career. Even today, my shifts in the emergency room are 24-hour shifts! From all of this, I can personally attest to the negative and powerful effects of sleep deprivation and the damage it can cause.

Sleep deprivation is one of the most harmful things you can do to your body. Without enough sleep, it can't heal, repair, or grow. Sleep deprivation leaves the body's immunity compromised and in a state of chronic stress and inflammation. This chronic stress state leads to a much earlier onset of common chronic diseases such as dementia, heart disease, diabetes, obesity, and high blood pressure. Sleep deprivation is probably the biggest risk factor for developing early-onset dementia and other cognitive and mood disorders.

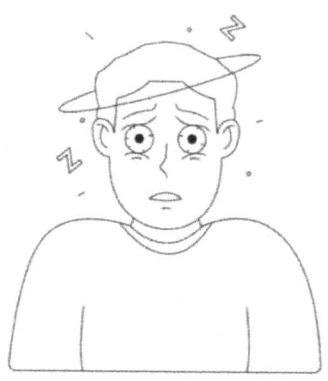

*Without enough sleep, your body can't heal,
repair or grow.*

For many years, scientists didn't understand the role sleep played in our lives. In the 1920s, the "father of American sleep research," Dr. Nathaniel Kleitman, began studying the cyclical nature of sleep, which led to today's study of sleep disorders such as sleep deprivation, sleep and circadian rhythms, and sleep and aging. Rapid eye movement (REM), one of the most important stages of sleep that occurs in deep sleep, wasn't discovered until 1953 by Kleitman's student, Dr. Eugene Aserinsky. Now we know that REM is a unique and essential part of the four sleep cycles that we move through during sleep (see section on The Sleep Stages). Today, we're continuing to learn about the link between good quality sleep and optimal health.[47]

Sleep involves many complex physiological functions that simply can't happen while we're awake. During sleep, our heart rate slows down, our blood pressure falls, our core body temperature decreases, and our digestive activity declines. Sleep is when the body goes to work repairing damaged tissues and forming new memories. When we sleep, our bodies clean up cellular waste, our brains are able to store new memories, and our immune system is strengthened. There are also some very important hormones that are released during sleep, including growth hormone, which can be thought of as an antiaging hormone of sorts that is responsible for cellular repair and growth.

Our hunger is controlled effectively through two hormones: leptin, a hormone that suppresses hunger, and ghrelin, which makes us feel hungry and helps signal the brain and gut when we should eat. Without sufficient sleep, the body's ability to regulate these hormones is disrupted and, as a result, so are our appetites. This is the main reason that you gain weight when you're sleep deprived.

Without good sleep the body's ability to regulate important hormones is disrupted and as a result so are our appetites. So, sleep deprivation often leads to weight gain.

Other important hormones affected by sleep include:

Cortisol, which normally peaks in the morning and then decreases in the late afternoon and evening, reaching its lowest levels during sleep. Cortisol is the main stress hormone that adapts the body to stress and affects many health factors, including mood, motivation, fear, blood pressure, blood sugar, and inflammation. If we don't get enough sleep, cortisol becomes chronically elevated, causing chronic stress, inflammation, and mood disorders, including chronic fatigue and poor focus and concentration

Melatonin, whose levels begin to rise in the evening to make us sleepy and which prepares the body and brain for sleep. Melatonin levels drop around 6:00 a.m., enabling us to wake up and begin our day.

The 5 Habits of Healthy People

The Five Stages of Sleep

In a full night's sleep (7.5–8.5 hours), our body naturally cycles through the five sleep stages approximately five times:

Stage 1: wakefulness;
Stage 2: light sleep;
Stage 3: deeper sleep;
Stage 4: very deep sleep; and
Stage 5: REM sleep.

The last and deepest sleep phase consists of REM sleep. In this stage our eyes move back and forth in response to our dreams. Each complete cycle of the five sleep stages lasts approximately 90 minutes, so in a seven- to nine-hour night of sleep, we will cycle through all five stages four to six times.

←——————————— 100% SLEEP CYCLE ———————————→

STAGE 1 (4-5%)	STAGE 2 (45-55%)	STAGE 3 (4-6%)	STAGE 4 (12-15%)	STAGE 5 (20-25%)
LIGHT SLEEP. MUSCLE ACTIVITY SLOWS DOWN. OCCASSIONAL MUSCLE TWITCHING.	BREATHING PATTERN AND HEART RATE SOWS. SLIGHT DECREASE IN BODY TEMPERATURE	DEEP SLEEP BEGINS. BRAIN BEGINS TO GENERATE SLOW DELTA WAVES.	VERY DEEP SLEEP. RHYTHMIC BREATHING. LIMITED MUSCLE ACTIVITY. BRAIN PRODUCES DELTA WAVES.	RAPID EYE MOVEMENT. BRAINWAVE SPEED UP AND DREAMING OCCURS. MUSCLES RELAX AND HEART RATE INCREASES. BREATHING IS RAPID AND SHALLOW.

TWO TYPES OF SLEEP

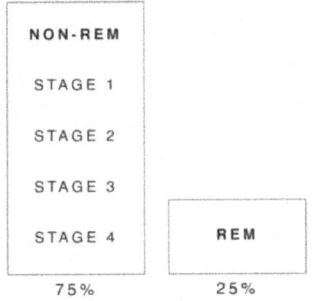

NON-REM

STAGE 1

STAGE 2

STAGE 3

STAGE 4   REM

75%   25%

The 5 Habits of Healthy People

It's Past Your Bedtime!

Today, we know that not sleeping enough or having chronically poor sleep can have deleterious effects. Not sleeping enough or getting low-quality sleep can affect our concentration, mood, and productivity because sleep is the time when our brains sort and store away the day's important memories, rebuild tissues, and release hormones that control our energy, mood, and focus.

Prior to the invention of indoor lighting, alarm clocks, smartphones, and nine-to-five work schedules, we were much more tuned in to our body's natural sleep-wake cycles. It turns out that what time you go to sleep and wake up makes a big difference in terms of the overall quality of your sleep and health.

Each of us has an internal alarm clock that is influenced by our hormones (i.e., cortisol and melatonin) and by our environment. Light is so crucial to sleep regulation that controlling it must be part of your sleep strategy!

Avoiding blue light from electronic devices and artificial indoor lighting is a good place to start. Using blue light–blocking glasses before bedtime sets your brain and body up to get a good night's sleep. Your sleep environment should be pitch black to the point that you cannot see anything, even when your eyes adjust after switching off the lights.

When our sleep suffers, our endocrine (hormonal) system also suffers and gets thrown out of whack.

This causes a decreased immune response and a decreased ability to regenerate cells and tissues. The cascade of temperature dysregulation, increased stress hormones, appetite imbalances, and increased inflammation that happen with lack of sleep are truly devastating. This is why keeping your sleep schedule as consistent as possible is so important.

How to Improve Your Sleep

A good night's sleep is also your key to productivity. Prior to settling into bed, here are some general recommendations for falling asleep faster and staying asleep longer:

Foods: Avoid eating high-calorie meals before bed, so your digestive system won't have to kick into overdrive before you go to sleep. If your body is using energy (and heating up) to digest food, it won't be cooling down for deep and REM sleep. Eating large, fatty meals before bedtime can also disrupt the release of the hunger-suppressing hormone, leptin, which can lead to food cravings during the day and can also affect the quality of restorative sleep.

Supplements: If you need help falling asleep easier and earlier, there are several supplements that can help you to adjust your sleep schedule. These include melatonin, valerian root, and cannabidiol oil (i.e., CBD oil derived from cannabis);

Napping: If you've missed an hour or two of sleep, napping during the day can help you catch up on missed cycles of sleep from the previous night.

Exercise: For optimal sleep, human performance and longevity expert Ben Greenfield recommends doing lower-intensity exercise such as walking, stretching, swimming, or yoga in the morning and harder, more vigorous exercise in the afternoon or early evening, being sure to finish at least three hours before bedtime.[48]

Environment: Make your bedroom a relaxing place to sleep by using calming essential oils, listening to soothing sounds, and finding activities that help you relax before bedtime. If you're stressed during the day, high cortisol levels can make it difficult to fall asleep and stay asleep throughout the night. Don't watch TV in the bedroom, and if you do, undo this habit, and start by getting the TV out of the bedroom!

Finding ways to improve and enhance the quality of sleep (and quantity) is a key step to dramatically improving your health. The National Sleep Foundation recommends that adults get seven to nine hours of quality sleep per night, and we agree. Fewer than seven hours per night has been shown to increase the risk of developing chronic diseases, and more than nine hours has no benefit. Try to keep your cycle of sleeping and wake times consistent.

Chapter 5

Habit #5: Five Keystone Health Measurements

W hen a patient comes in with undiagnosed high blood pressure, prediabetes, or diabetes, I find that many of these people had the disease (diabetes, metabolic syndrome) or the condition (high blood pressure) well before it was actually discovered. Most of these conditions develop over time and can go unnoticed for years especially when people go long periods of time without seeing their doctor or other health-care providers.

Over the years, I've learned that tracking five key measurements on an ongoing basis over time is much more effective than periodic "spot" checks at the doctor's office. This will help you to keep on top of things and detect any diseases early on. This makes it much easier to remedy and prevent much of the damage that these diseases cause when going undetected for long periods of time.

In the United States, the lack of focus and funding for preventive care has had devastating effects on our society. Preventive monitoring by tracking these measurements is crucial not only to diagnosing conditions early but also to living a long and healthy life.

The 5 Habits of Healthy People

You can practice preventative monitoring by tracking four keystone measurements. It will help you diagnose unhealthy conditions early so you can live a long and healthy life.

You can easily track these metrics at home and do a better job than your doctor at monitoring your health. There are widely available and cost-effective ways to measure these metrics, which I will recommend as we go through each of the measurements.

The 5 Habits of Healthy People

Keystone Measurement 1: Blood Pressure

Blood pressure is an indirect measure of how hard the heart has to work to circulate blood throughout the body. Having a healthy blood pressure means that your heart and circulatory system don't have to work harder than necessary. Maintaining a healthy blood pressure is one of the best things you can do to preserve heart, brain, and kidney health.

Having high blood pressure (also called hypertension) means that your heart is working harder than it should to pump blood. Over time, this causes the heart to overgrow, which is one of the main causes of heart failure (a.k.a. hypertrophic cardiomyopathy). Initially, there are no symptoms with high blood pressure, which is why it's referred to as the "silent killer." However, high blood pressure can wreak havoc on multiple organs, including the brain, heart, and kidneys well before it is actually diagnosed.

Healthy arteries and veins are flexible and can easily expand and contract. When blood pressure is high, it can damage the cells lining the arteries and veins, making them stiffer, inflamed, and atherosclerotic (plaque buildup), limiting blood flow and increasing the risk of stroke, heart attack, and irregular heart rhythms (arrhythmias).

As arteries stiffen and narrow, the heart must worker harder to supply enough blood to the tissues. Oftentimes, this will cause the left ventricle of the heart (the one doing most of the pumping) to enlarge to keep up with the work it must do to pump the blood. This is called left ventricular hypertrophy. As the heart eventually becomes overworked, it enlarges and, paradoxically, weakens, eventually leading to heart failure.

The 5 Habits of Healthy People

High blood pressure is no joke. It's important to know your numbers and track them regularly.

In the United States, an estimated one in three adults has high blood pressure, or about 100 million people, according to the CDC.[49] Of those people, only about half have their blood pressure controlled. Moreover, more kids and young people are at risk. An estimated 1.3 million youth have elevated blood pressure.[50]

What Are We Measuring?

A blood-pressure reading consists of two numbers. The top number is the systolic pressure, which is the pressure of the blood immediately following the contraction of the heart when blood is being pushed out of the heart into the circulatory system. The bottom number is the diastolic pressure, which is the pressure between the contractions of the heart when it is refilling with blood.

BLOOD PRESSURE CATEGORIES

BLOOD PRESSURE CATEGORY	SYSTOLIC mm Hg (upper number)		DIASTOLIC mm Hg (lower number)
NORMAL	LESS THAN 120	and	LESS THAN 80
ELEVATED	120-129	and	LESS THAN 80
HIGH BLOOD PRESSURE (HYPERTENSION) STAGE 1	130-139	or	80-89
HIGH BLOOD PRESSURE (HYPERTENSION) STAGE 2	140 OR HIGHER	or	90 OR HIGHER
HYPERTENSIVE CRISIS (consult your doctor immidiately)	HIGHER THAN 180	and/or	HIGHER THAN 120

* Referenced from American Heart Association.

The American Heart Association (AHA) includes healthy blood pressure ranges as a systolic reading of less than 120 mmHg over a diastolic reading of less than 80 mmHg.

Stage 1 of high blood pressure occurs when readings reach 130–139 mmHg (systolic) or 80–89 mmHg (diastolic). Lifestyle changes become more important at this stage, and medications may be considered. Lifestyle changes, including diet and exercise, should be attempted first.

Stage 2 occurs at 140/90 mmHg or higher, and medications and lifestyle changes will likely be prescribed by your doctor.

Readings higher than 180/120 mmHg indicate an urgent situation known as a hypertensive crisis.[51]

Having a healthy blood pressure starts with awareness. The first step in becoming more aware of your blood pressure is to take regular measurements on your own at home. Keep a record of these measurements. The easiest way to do this is to take a picture of them with your phone and then keep them in a separate file or as a "favorite" for easy access. Over time, a clear pattern will unfold and give you important information about your health, which can be shared with your doctor and other health-care providers.

Recommendations

Test your blood pressure twice a day for one week, once in the morning and once at night. If after one week, your numbers are within the normal range, change to testing twice a week (one day during the week and once on the weekend). If after one week, your numbers are elevated, continue measuring twice a day for one more week. If after the second week your numbers are still elevated at two different times, you can be pretty sure that you have high blood pressure, and we recommend seeing your doctor to be assessed. Be sure to take your readings in to show your doctor.

We recommend using an at-home automatic blood pressure cuff that fits around the upper arm (avoid the wrist cuffs as the accuracy is questionable). These can be purchased online or in many stores for under $50. You can also visit your local pharmacy and use their in-store blood pressure cuff. Take a photo with your phone or track the numbers in a journal or on your phone's Notes app.

Keystone Measurement 2: Fasting Blood Sugar

Fasting blood-sugar level is your blood-sugar value after not eating or drinking anything (except for water) for eight hours or longer. This is usually best checked first thing in the morning upon waking.

Tracking your fasting blood sugar is an indirect way to see how well your insulin is working and whether you're developing insulin resistance (which can indicate prediabetes that eventually can lead to type 2 diabetes). Remember, the role of insulin is to control sugar levels in the blood by transporting sugar out of the blood and into muscle and fat tissue for storage and later utilization by your muscles. Having high fasting blood-glucose levels over time means that your tissues aren't responding normally to the insulin, which is also called insulin insensitivity.

Generally, people diagnosed with type 2 diabetes had been living with it for some time before they are diagnosed. This is why tracking your own blood-sugar levels is so important.

What Are We Measuring?

For nondiabetics, fasting blood-sugar levels should be under 100 mg/dL, more specifically between 70 and 99 mg/dL. Fasting levels between 100 and 125 signal prediabetes. Fasting levels greater than 125 mg/dL signal type 2 diabetes.

For nondiabetics, blood-sugar levels should be less than 140 mg/dL two hours after eating. Fasting blood-sugar tests taken first thing in the morning should be under 100. A fasting blood-sugar level from 100 to 125 mg/dL is considered prediabetes. If it's 126 mg/dL or higher on three separate checks on three different days, that indicates diabetes.

BLOOD SUGAR BY THE NUMBERS

FASTING BLOOD GLUCOSE

▸ Normal   less than 100 mg/dL

▸ High Risk   100-125 mg/dL

▸ Diabetes   126 mg/dL or higher

HEMOGLOBIN A1c

▸ Normal   less than 5.7%

▸ High Risk   5.7-6.4%

▸ Diabetes   6.5% or higher

SOURCE: HARVARD HEALTH[52]

Earlier in this book, I discussed the hemoglobin A1C test. This test is a measure of the average blood-sugar levels in your blood over the past two to three months. Having a level of 6.5 percent or higher is a good indicator of diabetes. Levels between 5.7 percent and 6.4 percent are indications of prediabetes. Levels under 5.7 percent are considered normal.

Recommendations

When starting, we recommend testing your fasting blood-sugar levels once a day in the morning just after waking and before eating and drinking. Do this for seven days using an in-home blood sugar tester. If numbers are under 100 for a majority of the days, then continue measuring only once a week. If readings are over 100 for four or more days, then see a doctor to have your fasting blood sugar and hemoglobin A1C levels checked by them to determine if you are prediabetic or diabetic.

The 5 Habits of Healthy People

Keystone Measurement 3: Resting Heart Rate

Your resting heart rate is an important indicator of heart health and your heart's overall efficiency.

Your resting heart rate, also called your resting pulse, is the number of times your heart beats per minute while you are at rest. The more physically fit you are, the lower your resting heart rate will be. This is because a healthy and efficient heart will need to beat less often to do the same amount of work as a less efficient heart, because each pump sends out more blood with each contraction of the heart. A more efficient heart will also likely last longer than a heart that has to beat more often to do the same amount of work.

Resting heart rate can be affected by medications; stimulants like caffeine and nicotine; stress, which releases adrenaline and cortisol and causes your heart rate to rise; poor nutrition; inflammation; your activity levels; and the overall condition of your heart. Higher resting heart rates can indicate stress, fatigue, and poor conditioning. In general, a higher resting heart rate is an indication of a less fit or conditioned state. You can lower your resting heart rate by increasing your activity levels, improving your sleep, and improving your nutrition.

What Are We Measuring?

A normal resting heart rate can range between 60 and 90 beats per minute (bpm) for the average adult and can change, depending on fitness level, medication use, emotional state, body position (sitting or standing), age, and body size. The ideal range is between 50 and 70 bpm. A heart rate under 60 bpm when not due to a high fitness level (such as an athlete's) is called bradycardia, which can be a sign of more serious heart problem

The 5 Habits of Healthy People

WOMEN'S RESTING HEART RATE CHART

AGE	18 - 25	26 - 35	36 - 45	46 - 55	56 - 65	65+
ATHLETE	54 - 60	54 - 59	54 - 59	54 - 60	54 - 59	54 - 59
EXCELLENT	61 - 65	60 - 64	60 - 64	61 - 65	60 - 64	60 - 64
GOOD	66 - 69	65 - 68	65 - 69	66 - 69	65 - 68	65 - 68
ABOVE AVERAGE	70 - 73	69 - 72	70 - 73	70 - 73	69 - 73	69 - 72
AVERAGE	74 - 78	73 - 76	74 - 78	74 - 77	74 - 77	73 - 76
BELOW AVERAGE	79 - 84	77 - 82	79 - 84	78 - 83	78 - 83	77 - 84
POOR	85+	83+	85+	84+	84+	84+

MEN'S RESTING HEART RATE CHART

AGE	18 - 25	26 - 35	36 - 45	46 - 55	56 - 65	65+
ATHLETE	49 - 55	49 - 54	50 - 56	50 - 57	51 - 56	50 - 55
EXCELLENT	56 - 61	55 - 61	57 - 62	58 - 63	57 - 61	56 - 61
GOOD	62 - 65	62 - 65	63 - 66	64 - 67	62 - 67	62 - 65
ABOVE AVERAGE	66 - 69	66 - 70	67 - 70	68 - 71	68 - 71	66 - 69
AVERAGE	70 - 73	71 - 74	71 - 75	72 - 76	72 - 75	70 - 73
BELOW AVERAGE	74 - 81	75 - 81	76 - 82	77 - 83	76 - 81	74 - 79
POOR	82+	82+	83+	84+	82+	80+

Recommendations

We suggest testing your resting heart rate twice a day (once in the morning shortly after waking and once at night just before going to bed) using an activity tracker like a Fitbit® or pulse oximeter, which you clip to your finger (like the one that is used when you see your doctor). If the reading consistently runs high (over 90), schedule an appointment to discuss this with your doctor and keep an ongoing record of your resting heart rate over time so that you are aware of trends and patterns.

If you don't have an activity tracker or pulse oximeter, you can still get a reading the old-fashioned way. While standing or sitting still, place your first two fingers (not including your thumb) on the backside of your wrist on your thumb side and about one inch below where your wrist bends. Feel around until you can feel your heartbeat. Count the number of beats for 30 seconds. Multiply the number by two to get your resting heart rate in beats per minute.

Keystone Measurement 4: Percent Body Fat

When you hear the term "percent body fat," do you think of your body mass index (BMI)? Well, percent body fat and BMI are two completely different and unrelated measurements.

Percent body fat is a measure of the total amount of fat your body has as a percentage of your total weight. It's the ratio of total fat to total weight.

All of us have two types of fat on our bodies, essential and nonessential fat. Essential fat is crucial for reproductive health in women and serves to protect vital organs in the body. Nonessential fat is additional fat that can build up over time in our bodies and can cause serious health problems if levels get too high. A high percentage of fat is directly correlated with conditions such as metabolic syndrome, prediabetes, diabetes, and high blood pressure.

BMI, on the other hand, measures your height and weight to get a score based on the ratio of height and weight but does not take into account the kind of weight (muscle or fat) that is being used to determine the value. Because of this, BMI is an unreliable measure of health. Someone who is very muscular and lean (low percentage of body fat) can have a high BMI (implying that they are overweight), because BMI doesn't differentiate between muscle weight and fat weight.

Body mass index is an unreliable measure of health. It doesn't differentiate between muscle and fat. Percent body fat is better because it does.

The 5 Habits of Healthy People

Percent body fat is a very important measure to monitor over time, and maintaining a healthy body-fat percentage is a key factor in long-term health and longevity.

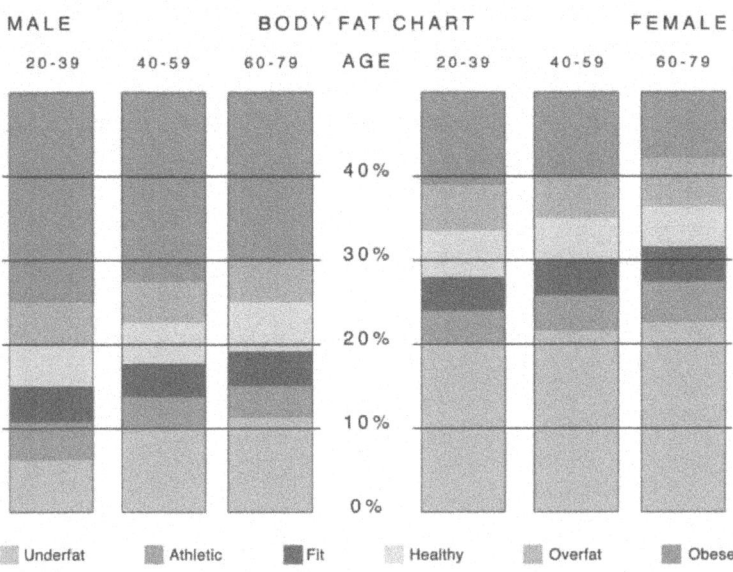

Recommendations

We suggest testing your percent body-fat once a month using a body fat monitor that uses bioelectrical impedance. We recommend you keep your percent body fat in the range of about 10–20 percent for men and about 20–30 percent for women for optimal long-term health.

Keystone Measurement 5: Hemoglobin A1C

Testing your hemoglobin A1C levels is important, as it gives you a bigger picture view of the general trends of your blood-sugar levels. Hemoglobin is the protein that carries oxygen in the blood. The more glucose (sugar) that is circulating in your blood stream, the more glucose will react with and bind to your hemoglobin. Once this happens, hemoglobin becomes known as hemoglobin A1C. The sugar molecules remain on the hemoglobin for the rest of the blood cell's life-span which is 120 days.

HEMOGLOBIN A1c

▸ Normal   less than 5.7%

▸ High Risk   5.7-6.4%

▸ Diabetes   6.5% or higher

Recommendations

Tracking your hemoglobin A1C levels should be done by your doctor as part of your regular blood testing. Doing this regularly will help screen for and detect diabetes or prediabetes early, making it easier to treat and often reverse. This test can also show you how well you are responding to treatment if you are diabetic. Testing your hemoglobin A1C levels is best done every three to six months. This test can also be done yourself by using one of the many online blood testing services such as https://www.wellnessfx.com/. There are also home test kits that can be purchased online for about $50 which will allow you to test your hemoglobin A1C four times.

Keep records of your Keystone measurements to show your doctor when you go. It's the first step to reclaiming control of your health.

Now that you've learned about the Five Keystone Health Measurements, I encourage you to make it a habit to test and keep track of these metrics regularly, set up a spreadsheet or a journal section so you can make notes, and remember to take it with you to show your doctor when seeing him or her. Doing this will give you a lot of insight into and provide you with a far better understanding of your own health than simply relying on what your doctor does. Being aware and acquiring knowledge are the most important steps in taking control of your health.

Goal-Directed Health

Goal-directed health is based on working toward specific health goals that are relevant and meaningful to you. Your goals can, and ideally will, include *The 5 Habits of Healthy People* that you just learned about, including the five health measurements we discussed in the previous section.

Setting goals for what we want to accomplish gives us clear, measurable parameters to work with.

For example, you might set the following health goals: I want to achieve a percent body fat of 15 percent, a resting heart rate of 60 bpm, a consistent average blood-pressure reading of 120/75 or less, and a fasting blood sugar that is consistently under 100.

Specific goals like these are much more powerful than vague goals such as "I want to lose weight, I want to look better, I want to feel better, and I want to eat better." By setting clear, measurable goals, we increase our chances of success because we have a clear understanding of what we are working toward.

The best way to achieve lasting results is to start with small steps. It builds confidence and enables you to see what's working for you and what's not so that you can change up the methods and tactics that don't work for you and find the ones that do.

The concept of goal-directed health is a concept developed out of my medical training and my own experiences of incorporating daily health and activity goals into my life. What has come out of this is *The 5 Habits of Healthy People* blueprint for achieving long-lasting health. By using goal-directed health and The 5 Habits blueprint, you too can make a true and lasting change in your life.

Chapter 6

My Own Health Journey and the Gravity Ball Story

At the beginning of this book, I described how the demands of my medical career had sabotaged my own health, causing me to gain weight and become unfit and unhealthy. I also told you how my father's injury made him unable to grip, which is what inspired me to develop a new way to do exercise called Grip-Free Resistance Exercise™. This new exercise method would allow people who had grip strength problems or other physical limitations with a way to exercise safely and effectively using weight.

The Development of Grip-Free Resistance Exercise and the Gravity Ball

In 2012, after a particularly long and grueling shift in the ER, I decided that I would quit my job for the purpose of taking back my health. I didn't know how I would survive or how I would get healthy again, but I knew I had to do it and that I had to start immediately at that moment, or I would end up sick, depressed, full of regrets, and dead at an early age!

One of the things that I began doing was using a medicine ball to exercise with each day, doing various exercises that I knew from watching my dad exercise and using my creativity to come up with my own exercises. The medicine ball was simple and easy to use. It was convenient, and I could use it in a small space.

Something that I didn't like about the medicine ball was that, in order to use it, you almost always had to have the ball between your two hands. To use it with one hand, you had to balance the ball in the palm of your hand and lift it while keeping your palm face up. I found this to be quite limiting, restrictive, and not a particularly fun way to exercise.

It occurred to me that the world needed a no-grip medicine ball that could be used with one hand and in any direction. This meant attaching it to the hands or the feet without the need to grip the ball while still benefiting from the additional force produced by the weight of the ball.

I believed that this concept of a new, improved, and highly versatile and functional medicine ball that could be thought of as the "Swiss Army Knife" of exercise balls could serve as the single piece of equipment that could provide everything the body needs to stay healthy, strong, and mobile.

To test the idea, I made various prototypes of the concept I had in my head. I turned my apartment into a workshop and began attaching straps, hooks, handles, and belts from old backpacks and bags to homemade medicine ball to produce handmade prototypes of what would eventually become the Gravity Ball.

The 5 Habits of Healthy People

I arranged the strap systems in a variety of ways to differently weighted balls that I made by filling old volley balls or soccer balls with sand. What I saw was something different, something that I had never seen before, something I knew I would enjoy using now and into the future, because it could adapt with me as my fitness levels changed.

I believe my Gravity Ball could become the "Swiss Army Knife" of medicine balls because it provides everything a body needs to stay healthy.

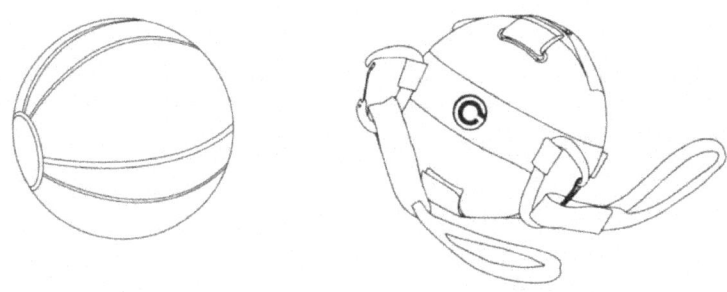

I also realized that my new-concept medicine ball would also benefit my dad and many people like him with grip-strength weakness, since they wouldn't need to grip it to use it. This inspired me to work on the concept that would eventually become the Gravity Ball.

After creating the initial prototype, I began using it daily. Whenever I would flip on the TV, I would reach for my Gravity Ball. I also modified my diet and started running again. Over time and with consistent effort, I was able to lose the extra 60 pounds that I had gained and have been able to keep it off for the last seven-plus years!

Origins of the Gravity Ball Method

The fitness industry has changed since the days I spent with my father in the gym. The traditional gym I remember was filled with intimidating iron equipment and lots of sweaty, grunting men. This gym environment works for some, but many of us have no desire to be in one and steer clear.

Other barriers to regular exercise include lack of time, motivation, uncertainty about how to exercise, and the lack of knowledge about which exercises are best to achieve long-term health goals.

Today's gyms are incorporating many new ways to exercise, including hybrid or mixed classes that blend various types of training methods or techniques to engage us in different ways. These new methodologies and mixed classes are exposing more people to exercise and expanding the fields of health, wellness, and fitness.

Gyms have also become hip, with mood lighting, piped music, and retail corners that sell fancy gym clothes and so-called health foods and supplements. Despite this transformation, much of the equipment used for resistance exercise has remained the same.

Despite watching my dad perform countless reps and sets in the gym when I was growing up, that way of exercising never made much sense to me. I was more inspired by the creative flow found in yoga, the centeredness of tai chi, and the impressive physical acts of gymnasts and acrobatics. I also enjoyed the zone or flow state that I felt when running or cycling. My own fitness journey has included long-distance running, cycling, and experimenting with yoga, as well.

Studying classical guitar in college taught me that the silence between the notes is as important as the music itself. As I developed the Gravity Ball Method, all these experiences and lessons combined with my medical training and self-study of anatomy served as strong influences that I would incorporate into the Gravity Ball Method.

My goal with the Gravity Ball Method was to incorporate all the benefits of resistance exercise in a way that was safe, effective, challenging, and fun. I wanted it to adapt to my mood and be easy to use in any setting at any time. The Gravity Ball Method has become my way of staying healthy, strong, flexible and mobile. I practice it every day, and as a result, I have been able to maintain a healthy weight and body-fat percentage by making it a habit.

Now I'm going to walk you through the principles of the Gravity Ball Method.

The 5 Habits of Healthy People

The Five Principles of the Gravity Ball Method

Five different principles are at work in the Gravity Ball Method™: Performing the exercises for a set amount of time (not reps or sets), time under tension, symmetry, balance and strength.

Timed

Once you pick up the Gravity Ball, the progression of exercise flows through concentric (muscle shortening), eccentric (muscle lengthening), and isometric (muscle is static) contractions that are held for a period of time without doing repetitions. This can be thought of as the Atlas principle based on the Greek myth that tells of the story of Atlas the Titan who was made by Zeus to forever hold the weight of the heavens never to rest.

Use a stopwatch, clock, or a countdown timer to track the amount of time you perform the various exercise sequences. They should be timed intervals of 10, 20, or 30 minutes at a time, totaling 30 minutes per day.

This means that, once you pick up the Gravity Ball, you do not put it down again until you finish the specified time you have set for that particular session.

This means that, once you pick up the Gravity Ball, you do not put it down again until you finish the specified time you have set for that particular session. Unlike most other weighted-exercise methods or programs, the focus is not on reps and sets. Instead, it's on going through different movements, poses, stretches, and exercises using correct technique and form with timed isometric poses and functional variations throughout various ranges of motion.

Time under Tension

In the Gravity Ball Method, you don't rest by putting the weight down; you rest by changing the pose, position, or movement so that a new group of muscles are working while the fatigued muscles are allowed to rest. This differs from doing repetitions and sets with rests in between. You move the Gravity Ball through different exercises (including using the "Up and Out" and "Down and In" method discussed below) to increase and decrease the difficulty of the exercise for a set period of time to complete the workout.

Symmetry

The Gravity Ball Method works on each side of the body separately so that imbalances and weaknesses are discovered and addressed to achieve symmetry throughout the body. This is done using functional movements that simulate common daily demands. The focus is on form rather than repetitions with the goal being to safely strengthen, stabilize, and align the major joints while increasing overall strength and minimizing joint wear and tear. The Gravity Ball Method utilizes exercises, poses, and movements that are highly functional and incorporate multiple major muscle groups into each exercise when possible.

Balance

Optimal body alignment is achieved through balance and conscious, purposeful movement. The Gravity Ball Method consciously and mindfully works on the balance center of the nervous system by focusing on movements and poses that increase mobility, stability, and balance. As you progress and the exercises become more difficult, the core becomes increasingly engaged. This is done with symmetric movements that utilize pushing, pulling, squatting, lunging, planking, and rotations.

Strength (using the "Up and Out" Principle)

The Gravity Ball Method can be changed and customized for anyone, from beginners to the advanced athlete. By using the principles of "Up and Out" and "Down and In," you can adjust the level of difficulty and the progression of the exercises. By moving the Gravity Ball "Up and Out," you intensify the level of core engagement and increase the efficiency of each exercise.

For example, holding the Gravity Ball further away from, or above, the body during a movement, pose, or exercise will increase the intensity and core engagement. As the weight moves further from the center of gravity, isometric and rotational forces increase core activation.

To decrease the intensity of the exercise or pose, bring the Gravity Ball "Down and In," closer to your center of gravity, as you perform the exercise.

The Gravity Ball Method combines backward, forward, and side-to-side movements into various movement patterns to target all the body's major muscle groups. It was designed to be a full-body strength-training and flexibility program for people who want to incorporate resistance exercise into their routine. The principles and exercises are designed to build strength, improve balance, achieve symmetry, and enhance musculoskeletal function. Exercises can be tailored to support each individual's particular needs and goals.

The 5 Habits of Healthy People

I spent many years developing and testing the exercises of the Gravity Ball Method with various Gravity Balls of different sizes and weights. The principles were inspired by the flexibility, symmetry, and stability of yoga as well as the strengthening and core work of Pilates, the creativity of acrobatics, and the benefits of weightlifting. The Gravity Ball Method of Grip-Free Resistance Exercise continuously engages the major muscle groups of the body as the body moves smoothly between one movement and the next.

Five Basic Movements of the Gravity Ball Method

The Gravity Ball Method incorporates:

1) Presses, which are pushes that involve bending at the elbow or at the knee;

2) Lifts, which involve lifting the weight away from you while keeping your arm or leg straight (no bending at elbow or knee);

3) Squats to strengthen the muscles supporting your hips, pelvis, spine, glutes, and knees;

4) Plank and plank variations, which are ideal for strengthening the stabilizing muscles along your core and spine; and

5) Lunges and lateral lunges, which have similar benefits as squats, but which incorporate a side-to-side element of balance and mobility training that many times is neglected in favor of backward and forward movements.

While practicing these exercises, strive to achieve symmetry between both halves of your body; this will reduce and oftentimes eliminate joint pains and muscular imbalances. As described above, work each side of the body separately so that the imbalances are found and over time focused on and corrected. This will help prevent injury, decrease or eliminate joint pains, and improve overall joint function.

The Major Joints

The Gravity Ball Method focuses on the following major joints: spine, shoulders, elbows, wrists, hips, knees, and ankles.

The 5 Habits of Healthy People

The shoulder joint is a ball-and-socket joint. Being the most mobile of all the joints, it is also the most injured. The shoulder joint can move in a complete circle, while still moving out, up, and back. Keeping the muscles of the rotator cuff and tendons surrounding the shoulder joint strong and balanced prevents potential injuries.

The knee joint (a hinge joint) is only designed to move out and back, like a door hinge. Knee joints are also regularly injured from wrong movements or imbalanced muscles or when the joint is twisted in a direction it's not designed to go.

The hip joints are also ball-and-socket joints that have a high degree of mobility, although less so than the shoulder because of the shape of the pelvis. They are a pivotal part of the body, and the location of many muscle attachment sites while serving as the middle point for the legs and the spine. It's very easy for the hips to be unbalanced, whether they are tilted forward, back, or to the side. When this happens, you can experience issues with your gait or pain in your back or knees.

Three Positions of Life

We spend our time each day lying down, sitting down, or standing. For this reason, the Gravity Ball Method uses all three positions of life.

Doing exercises in all three of these positions, you will strengthen the major muscle groups that you rely on throughout the day. This also gives you more flexibility to exercise wherever you are, like sitting at a desk or lying in bed. By making the most out of the time you have each day in a variety of environments, you can develop the habit of using the Gravity Ball anytime and anywhere.

The Gravity Ball is designed to do everything you need a complete exercise program to do while fitting nicely into your everyday life.

The 5 Habits of Healthy People

Regardless of your fitness level or prior exercise experience, people are using the Gravity Ball Method at home and in physical therapy clinics, including athletes and their trainers. Each day more people benefit from using the Gravity Ball in their daily routine or their training program.

As Charles Duhigg says in his book, *The Power of Habit*, a keystone habit can positively affect other things in your life without your having to take any further deliberate action. For example, exercising every day can lead to healthier eating, improved focus, improved productivity, and better sleep, all as a positive side effect of practicing the one keystone habit of exercising.

Daily resistance exercise using the Gravity Ball became a keystone habit for me. It's the reason I have been able to maintain a healthy weight and positive self-esteem over the years. By reshaping not just your body but your life with healthier habits, you will have more confidence, self-esteem, energy, and the ability to take charge of your life.

Closing Thoughts

Taking charge of your health isn't complicated, and it isn't hard to do. What's required and what does take time and effort is changing how you think and reevaluating what you have been told about health and exercise. Embracing *The 5 Habits of Healthy People* blueprint requires you to unlearn the things that don't provide a good return on your time investment. These simple but powerful habits are the key to taking back your health and staying in control of it for good.

Remember, each of us is different. For this reason, we may face unique health challenges that require a personalized plan to successfully face and overcome them. After working with patients for 15 years, I can confidently say that most people who have acquired one or more chronic conditions could have prevented them by simply following this simple five-step blueprint to healthy living.

I would like this book to serve as your guide to living a long and healthy life. It's time for physicians, health coaches, and other health professionals to change the landscape of health in our country by educating themselves, getting healthy, and leading by example.

Call to Action

After reading this book, I urge you to take the 5-month challenge to incorporate *The 5 Habits of Healthy People* into your life. A good goal is to incorporate at least one of the five habits into your routine each month over the next five months. Challenge your friends and family to join you. It's your right to own your health and not to have to rely on your doctor and the dysfunctional health-care system.

Become your own health-care advocate. After all, no one else cares about your health as much as you do.

So, go ahead; change your life. Remember, the best investments you can ever make are the investments you make in yourself.

APPENDIX

Evolution of the US Health-Care System

For much of history, you and your doctor had a one-on-one relationship that developed over time and grew with you and your family throughout life. Physicians knew their patient's names, and patients could call on them directly when needed. Major changes to the health care–delivery system, as we know it, began in the 1800s due in part to large technological and scientific advances as well as cultural developments and changes in leadership.

The health-insurance system that we are all familiar with has only existed during the last century and has encountered many struggles since health insurance was conceived. An early example of health insurance began in 1929, when Baylor University in Dallas offered its teachers 21 days of annual hospital care for a $6 monthly premium. In the 1920s, fewer than 20 percent of Americans had health insurance, and the costs of health care were beginning to rise. Private insurance companies began to realize that they could profit against the threat of illness and were beginning to offer coverage to healthier populations in order to cover reimbursements for those who needed the coverage. Other hospitals soon followed Baylor's example and began working with insurance companies to offer more health-coverage options.

In World War II, private employers began offering health insurance as a nontaxable fringe benefit valued at up to 5 percent of their pay.

This incentive was used to attract new workers at a time when wage limits were placed on employers due to the war. Unions became fans, and today nearly two-thirds of Americans still receive health-insurance coverage through their employers.

The decades following World War II experienced greater advancements in technology and science that made possible new lifesaving medications, vaccinations, and surgical techniques. As more people sought out these services, demand on the medical system increased. Hospital usage and costs rose in the 1940s and 1950s as a result of increased demand with a low supply.

In 1965, President Lyndon B. Johnson signed into law the legislation that established the Medicare and Medicaid programs which provided health-insurance coverage for Americans over the age of 65 and for low-income families, children, pregnant women, the elderly, and people with disabilities. With these two programs, groups who were previously ineligible for employer-sponsored health insurance were able to have access to coverage. Around this time, physicians also began to break out of the generalist-only role and began specializing in subspecialties within medicine.

In the 1980s physicians began working more closely with insurance companies, which had interwoven themselves into the hospital's payment structures. Hospitals and private corporations began collaborating, which led to the privatization of hospitals and insurance companies. Health Management Organizations (HMOs) and preferred provider organizations (PPOs) emerged to manage physician-patient interactions, allowing varying degrees of flexibility while also introducing more regulations into the field.

For many decades, there were attempts to offer universal coverage so that all Americans could receive health coverage, but the idea was labeled "socialized medicine" by some and wasn't supported by private companies and the organizations within medicine, which had the most to lose by changing the system. To this day, employer-based health-care coverage remains the prominent form of health care in the United States, and universal coverage remains a hotly contested topic.

Coverage Gaps of the Current Health Insurance System

Universal coverage is the provision of health-insurance coverage to all citizens of a nation simply based on citizenship. Many European countries as well as Japan and Singapore offer universal health-care coverage that is subsidized by the government and gives everyone access to coverage. Individuals who earn more in some countries have the option of purchasing private insurance that offers better access to services and shorter wait times to see specialists.

Currently the United States has a multipayer system, which means that insurance coverage comes from multiple sources (payers) including private-, public-, and voluntary-coverage options. Private coverage includes nongovernmental organizations and private companies that cover more than half of Americans (organizations such as Kaiser Permanente on the West Coast, Blue Cross, Aetna, and others). The remaining 40 percent of Americans receive public coverage, which includes Medicare and Medicaid, military coverage, and individual-market coverage.[53] Public (government) insurance covers close to one-third of Americans but accounts for *two-thirds of the nation's spending.*[54] This amount is expected to rise as the population ages and becomes more reliant on public-sponsored health care.

The Veteran's Affairs (VA) system and Medicare are examples of single-payer systems in the United States. Single-payer systems are single entities that pay for all health-care claims. Many countries have a single-payer system; however, the United States is much larger and more diverse both geographically and ethnically than these other countries, some of which have fewer than 10 million people. This is why many argue that a single-payer system would not be feasible for the United States.

The Affordable Care Act of 2016 is credited with reducing the uninsured population from about 47 million people to around 28 million. This was made possible by expanding Medicaid coverage in some states and by providing qualified individuals with assistance in purchasing private coverage. However, at the time of writing, the recent changes in the Affordable Care Act, and the possibility of repeal, leave many questions about the future of the health-care system in the United States.

Mostly, Medicaid is for the very poor, who have to qualify by being well below the official poverty line. Despite being adjusted for inflation, the federal poverty levels are far too low and exclude many struggling working-class Americans who do not qualify for state coverage because they earn more than the prescribed income limits. Yet they still struggle to survive high costs of living, particularly in high-cost states.

Medicaid coverage in 2018 includes people at or below 138 percent of the federal poverty level, which is $34,638 for a family of four. This excludes many people who earn $40,000, $50,000, or even higher, yet who still struggle. They must pay for their insurance premiums each month if not provided by their employer. These private health-care costs in the United States are also among the *highest in the world*. The high cost of coverage is the number-one reason uninsured adults cite for not having health insurance.

The 5 Habits of Healthy People

Without health insurance, access to lifesaving preventive services such as mammograms and annual physicals, naturally decreases, and as a result, when uninsured patients finally do seek help once they have fallen ill, their conditions are usually much worse. This increases the costs for both the individual and for society, compared with the costs of health screening and prevention. It's also an ethical dilemma for a modern, developed nation to have such a large number of uninsured people.

The 5 Habits of Healthy People

High Costs and Low Returns

Within the health-care system, the sad truth is that oftentimes, much of the money that is spent is wasted on unnecessary tests, questionable procedures, and overpriced medications that are not necessary or helpful and are sometimes dangerous. Why is this? Two big reasons for this are that when your physician orders multiple types of tests (blood, urine, radiology tests), it often makes the patient feel that something proactive or productive is being done. Additionally, these tests are quite expensive compared with the actual costs of manufacturing them, which make them a profitable revenue stream for multiple industries that provide the tests.

Another reason for extensive and expensive tests is to reduce liability on part of the physician in the case of a lawsuit; this practice of defensive medicine is a legitimate concern and barrier to providing high-quality health care.

Tests do have their place in medicine, but it is important to understand that simply doing more tests does not translate to better care.

The amount it costs to keep our health-care system afloat every year is astronomical. In 2014, the United States spent $3 trillion on health care, which breaks down to almost $10,000 ($9,923) per person. This is approximately 17.5 percent of the country's GDP, which is much more than any other developed nation spends on health care.[3] Shockingly, national spending on health care is expected to hit 20 percent of GDP by 2027.[55]

Some of the main drivers for these high costs are built into our relatively free market system. Countries with a single-payer system not only have subsidies on health-care costs but governments cap costs for procedures and pharmaceuticals. Our free-market system allows drug companies and insurers to control the markets and in turn charge whatever they want in order to continually raise their profit margins. This raises the prices for everyone involved in the system and ultimately places the final bill on the patient.

Despite having some of the most advanced drugs in the world, many Americans can't even afford prescription medications, which account for 16.7 percent of total personal health spending or $1,443 per capita.[56] Costs for procedures and high-tech diagnostic tests that can only be performed by your doctor also generate much more revenue for hospitals than routine, preventive services. High-volume, high-cost surgical procedures such as angioplasties, caesarean sections, and knee replacements are done much more in the United States than in other developed nations, oftentimes when the procedures are not even medically necessary or beneficial.[57]

In addition to not being trained or educated in topics relevant to keeping you healthy, doctors face many other pressures each day that patients don't see. They have a very limited amount of time with each patient (typically 10–15 minutes) and within that time period, they are expected to take a history; examine the patient; go over relevant testing, medication, and procedures; and diagnose, treat, prescribe, and educate the patient while completing the medical charting required for billing and compliance purposes. This oftentimes results in physicians diagnosing conditions that the patient doesn't actually have but that fit within the limitations prescribed by insurance companies to get reimbursed.

Medical billing was created to help standardize billing and treatment protocols for insurance companies. However, today it has become wasteful and inefficient. Version 10 of the *International*

Classification of Diseases (ICD-10) now contains 141,060 codes for medical diagnoses and procedures. This is a 712 percent increase over the 19,817 codes that were previously used in the ICD-9 version (more codes than contained in the *IRS handbook*!).[58]

The complexity of the billing system has become so excessive that it's now a barrier to providing proper care and is a major source of chronic stress to me and most other providers. Today physicians spend close to 25 percent of their resources on billing.[58] This is time not spent with patients, and as a result, the quality of patient care decreases while overhead increases and overall profits for health-care providers suffer. In order to make up for lost profits, physicians and other health-care providers need to see more patients in less time, which leads to poor experiences for the patient and a great amount of stress for the health-care provider. Because of this physician burnout, physician dissatisfaction and suicide are at an all-time high.

To top it off, deaths from medical errors ranks as the third leading cause of death in the United States.[59] This sad fact is due in part to low accountability in death certification reporting, and failing to teach physicians how to catch and correct errors. The sad fact is that, over the years, medical errors have remained stubbornly high. Despite extreme spending on pharmaceuticals, procedures, and costly health-care coverage, patients are still at risk of undue injury or death from medical errors.

It should be noted that the United States ranks well below many other Western European countries in terms of quality of life and has one of the lowest scores in terms of the quality of health-care delivery. Many people die every year in the United States due to not having access to adequate health care.[60]

For all these investments into technologically advanced treatments, we've found ways to lengthen our life-span at the cost of overcomplicating our health-care system and dramatically increasing the costs of health-care delivery. We've lost focus on teaching people and providing them with the basic tools and access to preventive health care to live longer with a higher quality of life. The current system is designed to profit off sickness. It's time for a new system that rewards healthy choices and incentivizes providers to keep people healthy throughout their lives.

The 5 Habits of Healthy People

For more information, visit TheHealthMD.com

For more information on the Gravity Ball and the Gravity Ball Method visit: GravityBall.com

[1] Duhigg, C. (2014). The power of habit: Why we do what we do in life and business. New York: Random House, LLC.

[2] Price, G., & Norbeck, T. (2018, April 9). U.S. health outcomes compared to other countries are misleading. Forbes. Retrieved from: https://www.forbes.com/sites/physiciansfoundation/2018/04/09/u-s-health-outcomes-compared-to-other-countries-are-misleading/#.

[3] Davis, W. (2012). Undoctored: *Why health care has failed you and how you can become smarter than your doctor*. New York: Rodale Wellness.

[4] Butler, S., Matthew, D., & Cabello, M. (2017, February 15). Re-balancing medical and social spending to promote health: Increasing state flexibility to improve health through housing. Brookings. Retrieved from: https://www.brookings.edu/blog/usc-brookings-schaeffer-on-health-policy/2017/02/15/re-balancing-medical-and-social-spending-to-promote-health-increasing-state-flexibility-to-improve-health-through-housing/.

[5] Pumping Iron. (n.d.). Retrieved from: https://en.wikipedia.org/wiki/Pumping_Iron.

[6] Schwarzenegger, A. (2019, January 2). Schwarzenegger: How I fought my way back to fitness. CNN. Retrieved from: https://www.cnn.com/2018/12/11/opinions/arnold-schwarzenegger-fitness-takes-work-dont-give-up/index.html.

[7] Department of Health & Human Services. (2018). Physical activity guidelines for Americans. 2nd edition [PDF File]. Retrieved

from: https://health.gov/paguidelines/second
edition/pdf/Physical_Activity_Guidelines_2nd_edition.pdf.

[8] Statistics about diabetes: Overall numbers, diabetes and prediabetes. (2018, March 22). Retrieved from: http://www.diabetes.org/diabetes-basics/statistics/.

[9] U.S. Department of Health and Human Services. (1985). Vital statistics of the United States: 1980 [PDF File]. Retrieved from: https://www.cdc.gov/nchs/data/vsus/mort80_2a.pdf.

[10] Eriksson, J., Taimela, S., Eriksson, K., Parviainen, S., Peltonen, J., & Kujala, U. (1997). Resistance training in the treatment of non-insulin-dependent diabetes mellitus. International Journal of Sports Medicine, 18(4):242–246. doi:10.1055/s-2007-972627.

[11] Eriksson, J., Tuominen, J., Valle, T., Sundberg, S., Sovijärvi, A., Lindholm, H., Tuomilehto, J., & Koivisto, V. (1998). Aerobic endurance exercise or circuit-type resistance training for individuals with impaired glucose tolerance. Hormone and Metabolic Research, 30(1):37–41. doi:10.1055/s-2007-978828.

[12] Poehlman, E. T., Dvorak, R. V., DeNino, W. F., Brochu, M., & Ades, P. A. (2000). Effects of resistance training and endurance training on insulin sensitivity in nonobese, young women: A controlled randomized trial. Journal of Clinical Endocrinology and Metabolism, 85(7):2463–2468. doi:10.1210/jcem.85.7.6692.

[13] Centers for Disease Control and Prevention. (2017). Heart disease facts. Retrieved from: https://www.cdc.gov/heartdisease/facts.htm.

[14] Leong, D.P., Teo, K.K., Rangarajan, S., Lopez-Jaramillo, P., Avezum A. Jr., Orlandini, A., Seron, P., Ahmed, S.H., Rosengren, A., Kelishadj, R., Rahman, O., Swaminathan, S., Iqbal, R., Gupta, R., Lear, S.A., Oquz, A., Yusoff, K., Zatonska, K., Chifamba, J., Iqumbor, E., Mohan, V., Anjana, R.M., Gu, H., Li, W., Yusaf, S. (2015). Prognostic value of grip strength: Findings from the Prospective Urban Rural Epidemiology (PURE) study. Lancet, 386(9990):P266–273. doi:10.1016/S0140-6736(14)62000-6.

[15] Epping, J. (2010). Weight training has unique heart benefits, study suggests. Medical News Today. Retrieved from: https://www.medicalnewstoday.com/articles/207417.php.

[16] McCartney, N. (1998). Role of resistance training in heart disease. Medicine & Science in Sports & Exercise, Oct(10 Suppl.):S396–402. Retrieved from: https://www.ncbi.nlm.nih.gov/pubmed/9789866.

[17] Centers for Disease Control and Prevention. (2019). High blood pressure. Retrieved from: https://www.cdc.gov/bloodpressure/index.htm.

[18] Morais, P.K., Campbell, C.S., Sales M.M., Motta, D.F., Moreira, S.R., Cunha, V.N., Benford, R.E., Simoes H.G. (2011). Acute resistance exercise is more effective than aerobic exercise for 24h blood pressure control in type 2 diabetics. Diabetes & Metabolism. 37(2):112–117. doi:10.1016/j.diabet.2010.08.008.

[19] Moeini, M., Salehi, Z., Sadeghi, M., Kargarfard, M., & Salehi, K. (2015). The Effect of Resistance Exercise On Mean Blood Pressure In Patients Referring to Cardiovascular Research Centre. Iranian Journal of Nursing and Midwifery Research. 20(4):431–435. doi:10.4103/1735-9066.160999.

[20] Mann, S., Beedie, C., & Jimenez, A. (2013). Differential Effects of Aerobic Exercise, Resistance Training and Combined Exercise Modalities on Cholesterol and the Lipid Profile Review, Synthesis and Recommendations. Sports Medicine (Auckland, N.Z.). 2014; 44(2): 211–221. doi:10.1007/s40279-013-0110-5.

[21] American Heart Association. (2018). Strength and resistance exercise. Retrieved from: https://www.heart.org/en/healthy-living/fitness/fitness-basics/strength-and-resistance-training-exercise.

[22] American Cancer Society. (2014). Physical activity and the cancer patient. Retrieved from: https://www.cancer.org/treatment/survivorship-during-and-after-treatment/staying-active/physical-activity-and-the-cancer-patient.html.

[23] ABC Science. (2016, May 10). Exercise & cancer | How targeted exercise can help fight cancer [Video File]. Retrieved from: https://www.youtube.com/watch?v=ffgAVrANmS4.

[24] Bushak, L. (2015, August 11). The stress of severe pain: 11% of Americans suffer from chronic pain, NIH states. Medical Daily. Retrieved from: https://www.medicaldaily.com/stress-severe-pain-11-americans-suffer-chronic-pain-nih-states-347292.

[25] Shanmugam, V.K., Couch, K.S., McNish, S., & Amdur, R.L. (2017). Relationship between opioid treatment and rate of healing in chronic wounds. Wound Repair and Regeneration: The International Journal of Tissue Repair and Regneration, 25(1): 120–130. doi:10.1111/wrr.12496.

[26] Chronic pain research delves into the brain. (2014, March 12). University of Adelaide. Retrieved from: https://www.adelaide.edu.au/news/news69222.html.

[27] Geneen, L.J., Moore, R.A., Clarke, C., Martin, D., Colvin, L.A., Smith, B.H. (2017). Physical activity and exercise for chronic pain in adults: An overview of Cochrane Reviews. Cochrane Database of Systemic Reviews, 2017 Jan 14;1:CD011279. doi: 10.1002/14651858.CD011279.pub2.

[28] O'Connor, P. J., Herring, M. P., & Carvalho, A. (2010). Mental health benefits of strength training in adults. American Journal of Lifestyle Medicine, 4(5):377–396. doi:10.1177/1559827610368771.

[29] Strickland, J., & Smith, M. (2014). The anxiolytic effects of resistance exercise. Frontiers in Psychology, 5:753. doi:10.3389/fpsyg.2014.00753.

[30] Kandel, E. (2016, May 6). How exercise improves brain function. U.S. News & World Report. Retrieved from: https://health.usnews.com/health-news/patient-advice/articles/2016-05-06/how-exercise-improves-brain-function.

[31] Kraschnewski, J.L., Sciamanna, C.N., Poger, J.M., Rovniak, L.S., Lehman, E.B., Cooper, A.B., Ballentine, N.H., Ciccolo, J.T. (2016). Is strength training associated with mortality benefits? A 15 year cohort study of US adults. Preventive Medicine, 87:121–127. doi:10.1016/j.ypmed.2016.02.038.

[32] Dalleck, L., & Kravitz, L. The history of fitness. University of New Mexico. Retrieved from: https://www.unm.edu/~lkravitz/Article%20folder/history.html#Anchor-2821.

[33] Illinois innovators: Thomas Cureton Jr., the father of physical fitness [Video File]. [Illinois1867]. (2012, July 17). Retrieved from: https://www.youtube.com/watch?v=9gdAHC7qq70.

[34] Hevesi, D. (2009, November 7). Jeremy Morris, who proved exercise is heart healthy, dies at 991/2. New York Times. Retrieved from: https://www.nytimes.com/2009/11/08/health/research/08morris.html.

[35] Heffernan, C. (2015, June 15). Born to run: The origins of America's jogging craze. Physical Culture Study. Retrieved from: https://physicalculturestudy.com/2015/06/15/born-to-run-the-origins-of-americas-jogging-craze/.

[36] Anderson, C. The fitness industry: Through the years. Shape. Retrieved from: https://www.shape.com/fitness/fitness-industry-through-years.

[37] Berry, J. (2019, January 21). What to know about essential amino acids. Medical News Today. Retrieved from: https://www.medicalnewstoday.com/articles/324229.php.

[38] Greenfield, B. The big fat surprise. Why butter, meat and cheese belong in a healthy diet (& What they don't tell you about the mediterranean diet) [Audio File Transcript]. Retrieved from: https://bengreenfieldfitness.com/transcripts/transcript-the-big-fat-surprise-why-butter-meat-and-cheese-belong-in-a-healthy-diet/.

[39] U.S. Food & Drug Administration. (n.d.). Trans fat. Retrieved from: https://www.fda.gov/food/food-additives-petitions/trans-fat.

[40] Greger, M. (2015, May 1). Are organic foods safer? [Video File]. Retrieved from: https://nutritionfacts.org/video/are-organic-foods-safer/.

[41] Dirty Dozen™. (n.d.). EWG's 2019 shopper's guide to pesticides in produce™. Retrieved from: https://www.ewg.org/foodnews/dirty-dozen.php 7.

[42] Gunter, M.J., Murphy, N, Cross, A.J., Dossus, L, Dartois, L, Fagherazzi, G, Kaaks, R, Kühn, T, Boeing, H, Aleksandrova, K, Tjønneland, A, Olsen, A, Overvad, K, Larsen, S.C., Redondo Cornejo, M.L., Agudo, A, Sánchez Pérez, M.J., Altzibar, J.M., Navarro, C, Ardanaz, E, Khaw, K.T., Butterworth, A, Bradbury, K.E., Trichopoulou, A, Lagiou, P, Trichopoulos, D, Palli, D, Grioni, S, Vineis, P, Panico, S, Tumino, R, Bueno-de-Mesquita, B, Siersema, P, Leenders, M, Beulens, JWJ, Uiterwaal, CU, Wallström, P, Nilsson, LM, Landberg, R, Weiderpass, E, Skeie, G, Braaten, T, Brennan, P, Licaj, I, Muller, D.C., Sinha, R, Wareham, N, Riboli, E. (2017, August 15). Coffee drinking and mortality in 10 European countries: A multinational cohort study. Annals of Internal Medicine. 167(4):236–247. doi:10.7326/M16-2945.

[43] Greenfield, B. 63 cups of coffee a day & more: Five simple things you can do to live a longer, healthier life [Audio File]. Retrieved from: https://bengreenfieldfitness.com/podcast/anti-aging-podcasts/live-a-longer-healthier-life-podcast-with-dr-sanjiv-chopra/.

[44] Greenfield, B. 23 years of suckin' down coffee: Tips, tricks & hacks I've discovered for getting the most out of one of the safest superfoods that exists. Retrieved from: https://bengreenfieldfitness.com/article/coffee-tips-tricks-hacks-or-getting-the-most-out-of-coffee/.

[45] Ferraro, P. M., Taylor, E. N., Gambaro, G., & Curhan, G. C. (2013). Soda and other beverages and the risk of kidney stones. Clinical Journal of the American Society of Nephrology, 8(8):1389–1395. doi:10.2215/CJN.11661112.

[46] Oregon Health & Science University. (2013, December 17). Study: Moderate alcohol consumption boosts body's immune system. Retrieved from: https://www.eurekalert.org/pub_releases/2013-12/ohs-sma121713.php.

[47] A brief history of sleep research. (1999, February 3). Retrieved from: https://web.stanford.edu/~dement/history.html.

[48] Greenfield, B. (n.d.). Module 4: Sleep—the missing link for better brains. In KionU 2019 Program [Presentation Slide]. Retrieved from: https://kionu.getkion.com/.

[49] Centers for Disease Control and Prevention. (2019, February 13). High blood pressure. Retrieved from: https://www.cdc.gov/bloodpressure/index.htm.

[50] Centers for Disease Control and Prevention. (2018, July 18). High blood pressure during childhood and adolescence. Retrieved from: https://www.cdc.gov/bloodpressure/youth.htm.

[51] American Heart Association. (2017, November 30). Understanding high blood pressure. Retrieved from: https://www.heart.org/en/health-topics/high-blood-pressure/understanding-blood-pressure-readings.

[52] Harvard Health. (2015). Rising blood sugar: How to turn it around [Online image]. Retrieved May 30, 3019 from

https://www.health.harvard.edu/diabetes/rising-blood-sugar-how-to-turn-it-around

[53] Two new federal surveys show stable uninsured rate. Health Affairs Blog, September 13, 2018. doi:10.1377/hblog20180913.896261.

[54] Syrop, J. (2016, February 2). Federal government funds two-thirds of healthcare costs, study finds. *American Journal of Accountable Care.* Retrieved from: https://www.ajmc.com/newsroom/federal-government-funds-two-thirds-of-healthcare-costs-study-finds-.

[55] National Health Expenditure Projections 2018–2027. (n.d.). Retrieved from: https://www.cms.gov/Research-Statistics-Data-and-Systems/Statistics-Trends-and-Reports/NationalHealthExpendData/Downloads/ForecastSummary.pdf.

[56] Price, G., & Norbeck, T. (2018, April 9). U.S. health outcomes compared to other countries are misleading. *Forbes.* Retrieved from: https://www.forbes.com/sites/physiciansfoundation/2018/04/09/u-s-health-outcomes-compared-to-other-countries-are-misleading/#f5a13ae12325.

[57] Kamal, R., & Cox, C. (2018, May 8). How do healthcare prices and use in the U.S. compare to other countries? Retrieved from: https://www.healthsystemtracker.org/chart-collection/how-do-healthcare-prices-and-use-in-the-u-s-compare-to-other-countries/#item-the-u-s-averages-fewer-angioplasty-and-more-bypass-surgeries-than-most-comparable-countries_2018.

The 5 Habits of Healthy People

[58] Price, G., & Norbeck, T. (2013, November 5). Healthcare is turning into a industry focused on compliance, regulation rather than patient care. *Forbes*. Retrieved from: https://www.forbes.com/sites/physiciansfoundation/2013/11/05/healthcare-is-turing-into-an-industry-focused-on-compliance-regulation-rather-than-patient-care/#7b53df3c2e3c.

[59] Study suggests medical errors now third leading cause of death in the U.S. (2016, May 3). *Johns Hopkins Medicine*. Retrieved from: https://www.hopkinsmedicine.org/news/media/releases/study_suggests_medical_errors_now_third_leading_cause_of_death_in_the_us.

[60] Radcliff, B. (2018, July 9). The US ranks last in health care system performance. Retrieved from: https://www.psychologytoday.com/us/blog/the-economy-happiness/201807/the-us-ranks-last-in-health-care-system-performance.

The 5 Habits of Healthy People

Made in USA - Kendallville, IN
80264_9781733151207
08.29.2022 1419